CS Checklists

Portable Review for the USMLE Step 2 CS (Clinical Skills Exam)

CS Checklists

Portable Review for the USMLE Step 2 CS (Clinical Skills Exam)

Second Edition

Jennifer K. Rooney, MD
Clinical Instructor
St. George's University
Grenada, West Indies

Reviewed by

Patrick Rooney, MD (Hons.), FRCP (Glasgow and Edinburgh) FACP
Department Chair of Clinical Skills
St. George's University
Grenada, West Indies

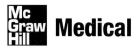

New York Chicago San Francisco Lisbon London Madrid Mexico City Milan
New Delhi San Juan Seoul Singapore Sydney Toronto

The *McGraw·Hill* Companies

CS Checklists: Portable Review for the USMLE Step 2 CS (Clinical Skills Exam), Second Edition

1 2 3 4 5 6 7 8 9 0   DOC/DOC   0 9 8 7

ISBN-13: 978-0-07-148823-5
ISBN-10: 0-07-148823-5

This book was set in Palatino by Techbooks.
The editor was Catherine A. Johnson.
The production supervisor was Phil Galea.
Project management was provided by Techbooks.
RR Donnelley was printer and binder.

This book is printed on acid-free paper.

Library of Congress Cataloging-in-Publication Data
Rooney, Jennifer K.
    CS Checklists : portable review for the USMLE Step 2 CS (clinical skills exam)/
Jennifer K. Rooney; reviewed by Patrick Rooney. – 2nd ed.
        p. ;   cm.
    ISBN-13: 978-0-07-148823-5 (soft cover : alk. paper)
    ISBN-10: 0-07-148823-5
1. Physical diagnosis–Examinations, questions, etc. 2. Medical history taking–
Examinations, questions, etc. 3. Diagnosis, Differential–Examinations, questions, etc.
4. Physicians–Licenses–Examinations–Study guides. I. Title. II. Title: Portable
review for the USMLE Step 2 CS (clinical skills exam).
    [DNLM: 1. Clinical Medicine–Case Reports. 2. Clinical Medicine–Examination
Questions. WB 18.2 R777ca2007] RC76.R66 2007 616.07′51076–dc22
                                                                                    2006034770

Contents

INTRODUCTION

The Clinical Skills Examination (CSE) is designed to assess the examinee's ability to interact with patients, obtain a history, and perform a physical examination. The examinee must be able to inform patients of findings, discuss potential diagnoses, and explain any work-up which he or she recommends. The ability to communicate the information gathered to colleagues and to the patient is also assessed. The examination is also used to assess proficiency in the English language.

The examination consists of 11 or 12 stations. At each station, the examinee is expected to obtain a history and may have to perform a physical examination. He/she then has to record the findings as well as provide a differential diagnosis and suggested follow-up for the patient. Each station starts with an examinee instruction sheet. The sheet contains general information about the patient (name, age, gender, reason for consult, and vital signs). Each instruction sheet will have a brief outline of what is expected of the examinee at the station. For example, the outline of what is expected on the instruction sheet may appear as follows:

1. Obtain a focused history
2. Perform a relevant physical examination
3. Discuss any pertinent findings with the patient

The examinee has approximately 15 minutes to obtain the history and perform the physical examination (if required), followed by 10 minutes to record the findings, the differential diagnosis, and the follow-up for the patient. The examinee also may also be required to provide some feedback and counseling to the patient during the initial 15 minutes. Each station will have all the necessary equipment (tongue depressors, eye charts, gloves, etc.) available for the examinee. Some of the stations may be telephone stations. In these stations, a telephone and a phone number will be provided and the examinee will be have to obtain a history over the phone and provide appropriate advice and counseling to the patient. Some stations may involve a child or an elderly patient who is not present. The interaction will be with the caregiver. The total duration of the examination is 7–8 hours, including intermittent short breaks and a lunch break.

The examination uses standardized patients who are individuals trained to portray real patients (both by history and by physical examination). The standardized patient responds to questions asked by the examinee and participates in a physical examination. The standardized patients have extensive training and use specific checklists and rating scales to evaluate the examinee. The examination may also be observed by physicians who may assess the examinee's performance and review the final score received by the examinee, ensuring the fairness of the scoring done by the standardized patient. The standardized patient will remain in role throughout the examination. The examinee should not attempt to interact/converse with the standardized patient outside of the patient role.

For many years foreign medical students were required to take the Clinical Skills Assessment Examination (CSA). In a move to make certification requirements the same for US medical school graduates and international medical graduates, the National Board of Medical Examiners made the new USMLE Step 2 CS (Clinical Skills) component a requirement for all medical students seeking licensure. The information included in this handbook has been gathered from both recent foreign graduates who have taken the CSA and from very recent graduates who have taken the Step 2 CS. Common patient clinical presentations from the examination have been included as well as checklists, physical examination findings, differential diagnosis, follow-up, and brief case reviews for each patient clinical presentation. The cases which may be presented during the examination are generally representative of the core clerkships of medical schools in the United States. These include internal medicine, pediatrics, surgery, obstetrics/gynecology, psychiatry, and family medicine.

The USMLE Step 2 CS was launched in 2004. The first class required to take it was the graduating class of 2005. Passing scores in the USMLE Step 1 and Step 2 CK, along with a passing score on the Step 2 CS, is required for all graduates prior to entering a residency program in the United States. Candidates may take Step 1, Step 2 CK, and the Step 2 CS in any order, but must pass all of them prior to taking Step 3.

As of the time of this book's publication, the Step 2 CS is currently being administered at the following sites: Philadelphia, Atlanta, Los Angeles, Chicago, and Houston. The cost of taking the examination is $1200.00. The examinee must also consider the additional cost of travel to one of these centers and possibly the cost of overnight accommodation near the center also.

Preparing for the USMLE Step 2 CS

GENERAL INFORMATION

It is recommended that you arrive at the examination center with enough time prior to the start of your examination to sit and relax for a few minutes. The CSE is a lengthy, stressful examination, and so take a few minutes to mentally prepare prior to the start of your session.

It is also recommended that you review all of the checklists provided in this handbook as well as practice patient write-ups prior to the day of the examination.

At each patient station, you will wait outside the examination room door, and an announcement will tell you when to begin the patient encounter. Start by reading the examinee instruction sheet provided on the door, knock, and then enter the room.

Important Tips

- Dress appropriately (smart, comfortable, professional attire).
- If possible, locate the examination center one day prior to your examination, or earlier on the day of the examination, so as to avoid any unnecessary stress in trying to find the center at the time of the examination.
- Arrive early for your examination.
- Bring your stethoscope and your white lab coat with you (all other equipment will be provided to you).
- Bring your scheduling permit and an unexpired government issued form of identification.
- A light meal will be provided during the examination; however, you may wish to bring your own lunch with you (no refrigeration is available at the testing site).
- Once you have entered the secure testing site, you will not be permitted to leave until the examination is completed.
- You will be given an orientation/introduction session prior to the start of the examination. Listen carefully to the instructions given to you.

▓ A demonstration of the equipment available during the examination will be given during the orientation session.

▓ The orientation video is available on the USMLE Web site if you would like to view it prior to your examination day.

▓ Carefully read the examinee instruction sheet prior to entering the room. A copy of the sheet will be provided in the room for further reference.

▓ Be sure to introduce yourself to the patient at each station. Be honest about yourself. If you are a medical student, introduce yourself as such. If you are already a physician, introduce yourself as such.

▓ Vital signs will be provided to you prior to the start of the patient encounter. You may choose to repeat the vitals if you feel that it is necessary, for example, in the case of a patient with hypertension. Consider the vitals provided on the examinee instruction sheet as the actual vital signs of the patient as you write up the case.

▓ *Always* elicit the patient's

   Name

   Age

   Address

   Occupation

   Presenting complaint

   Some of these details may be provided to you on the patient information sheet, and if so do not request them again during the interview. It may be useful to confirm the information at the start of the interview, for example, "You are Ms Smith. Is that correct?"

▓ Establish and maintain eye contact with the patient.

▓ Minimize physical barriers; for example, if there is a desk in the room, have the patient sit at the side of the desk rather that in front of the desk.

▓ Begin the patient interview with open-ended questions. Allow the patient to respond to the questions without interruption. Avoid multiple questions. Sequence questions appropriately using recap/summary technique.

▓ Indicate to the patient that you are paying attention by using nonverbal cues as well as verbal cues. Show empathy to the patient verbally and by posture and body language. Use echoing (repeating the last word or phrase used by the patient) to let the patient know that you are listening and that you are concerned. Use active continuers such as "Go on," "I hear you," and "Tell me more."

- Always acknowledge the patient's feelings and concerns.
- Try to avoid the use of medical or technical terms and always try to ascertain that the patient understands the terms that you are using.
- Prior to the physical examination, explain to the patient what you are planning to do before you actually start the examination.
- Always wash your hands before and after any physical examination of the patient.
- Offer the patient assistance in both getting on and off the examination table.
- If the patient is lying on the examination table, be sure to pull out the leg support.
- Never examine the patient through clothing. However, remember to be sensitive to the patient's privacy.
- Rectal, pelvic, genitourinary, female breast, and corneal reflex examinations should not be performed during the examination. If you think that any of these examinations is an important diagnostic step in the case, include it in the follow-up.
- Be aware of the fact that the standardized patients are examined repeatedly throughout the course of the day. Try to be as gentle as possible while doing any aspect of the physical examination.
- Physical examination checklists in this handbook generally include only components of the physical examination relevant to the patient clinical presentation given. If time permits, other parts of the complete examination may be performed.
- At the end of each patient station, explain to the patient your initial diagnostic impressions. The patient may wish to ask questions at some point during the session. Be aware of this and be ready to answer any questions that they may have. You should also inform the patient of any follow-up you would like to have done, for example, lab work, X-rays, and so on. Inform the patient of any changes in their lifestyle you would like him/her to attempt and when the most appropriate follow-up visit should take place.
- Remember, your write-up must be legible and should include positive findings in the history and the physical examination as well as negative findings. The write-up may be done by hand or typed on a computer.
- Use only those abbreviations which you are certain are acceptable. If you are unsure whether an abbreviation is acceptable, do no use it, instead write it out in full. There may be a list of acceptable abbreviations at the examination site for your use.

- The differential diagnosis should be written in order of the most likely diagnosis to the least likely diagnosis.
- Please note that during the actual examination you will be required to list five or fewer differential diagnoses as well as list five or fewer follow-up plans. The cases presented in this book allow for more differential diagnosis and follow-up plans.
- The follow-up should include all further physical examination (e.g., pelvic examination) and testing that is appropriate.
- Drugs, referrals, surgery, consults, and therapeutic procedures are not permitted as part of the follow-up.
- Some of the cases presented in this book do not include physical diagnosis checklists or findings. For these cases, assume that the physical examination findings are normal and therefore will not affect the differential diagnosis or the follow-up.

COMPONENTS OF A COMPLETE HEALTH HISTORY

A complete history should include all of the following:
1. Chief complaint
2. History of the presenting illness
3. Medical history
4. Surgical history
5. Allergies
6. Medications
7. Obstetric/gynecology history
8. Social history
9. Family history
10. Review of systems

Chief Complaint

The chief complaint is what prompted the patient to seek medical care. Try to allow the patient to tell you in his/her own words what the problem is. Open-ended questions are particularly useful for obtaining the chief complaint.

History of the Presenting Illness

This covers the presenting illness from the onset of the symptoms. Allow the patient to relay the events/onset of each symptom as it occurred. After allowing the patient to summarize the history of the illness, direct questions may be useful to obtain any further information.

Fully investigate the principal symptoms with descriptions of

1. onset
2. location
3. character
4. duration
5. frequency
6. severity
7. aggravating factors
8. relieving factors
9. medications taken to relieve symptoms and their effects
10. associated symptoms
11. the impact on the patient (self, family, occupation)

Medical History

The medical history includes all illnesses that the patient currently has as well as illnesses that he/she has had in the past, which have since resolved, including childhood illnesses. The dates of past illnesses should be established and recorded as well as the dates of onset of any current illnesses. An immunization history should also be included here.

Past Surgical History

This includes *all* surgeries and the dates of each surgery. Ask specific questions regarding the surgeries, if necessary. For example, elicit the reason the patient had the surgery done, whether it was a successful operation, and any complications encountered following the surgery.

Allergies

Inquire about all drug allergies. Also establish the exact reaction that occurred when the patient took the specific medication. Inquire about environmental and food allergies.

Medications

Inquire about all medications and their doses that the patient is currently taking. Ask the patient why he/she takes a specific medication, especially if you are unfamiliar with the medication and its uses. Also inquire about medications taken by the patient in the past.

Obstetric/Gynecology History

Inquire about the patient's menstrual cycle and establish the following:

- Is it regular?
- How often does menstruation occur?
- How long does it typically last?
- Does the patient have very heavy periods or very painful periods?
- When was the last menstrual period?
- What age was menarche?
- What age was menopause (if relevant)?

Inquire about the patient's obstetric history and establish the following:

- How many pregnancies has the patient had?
- What was the outcome of each pregnancy?
- What was the date of each pregnancy?
- What method of birth control does the patient currently use, if any?

Inquire about the patient's sexual history and establish the following:

- Is the patient currently sexually active? If so, with how many partners?
- What type of protection is the patient using against sexually transmitted diseases?
- Has the patient ever been diagnosed with a sexually transmitted disease?
- Female

  When was the last pelvic examination done?

  When was the last papanicolaou (pap) smear taken?

  Has the patient ever had any abnormal pap smears? If so, what was the treatment or the follow-up required?

▨ Male

   Is the patient able to achieve and maintain an erection?

   Is ejaculation normal?

   What was the date of the last physical examination (including examination of the genitalia)?

Social History

The social history should include the patient's family life, employment situation, and daily habits. Elicit the patient's religion (or lack of religious belief) and if practiced currently. A history of alcohol use, cigarette use, and drug use should also be included. Be sure to inquire as to how much, how often, and for what period of time the patient has been using each substance. Other risk behaviors (e.g., hang gliding, SCUBA diving) should also be addressed as well as inquiring about diet and exercise.

If you suspect that the patient has a problem with alcohol abuse, the CAGE questions can be asked. These include the following:

1. Have you ever felt the need to *cut down* on your drinking?
2. Have you ever felt *annoyed* when someone mentions your drinking or suggests that you cut down?
3. Have you ever felt *guilty* about your drinking or something that you did while under the influence?
4. Have you ever needed an *eye opener*?

Family History

Inquire about the patient's spouse or partner, parents, siblings, and children. Take note of any medical problems in the family. Pay particular attention to common disorders with an increased contact risk (e.g., tuberculosis) or an increased inherited risk (e.g., diabetes mellitus or hypertension).

Review of Systems

Following completion of the components of the history, a review of systems can be a useful tool for picking up any symptoms that may not have been mentioned by the patient previously.

The review of systems should consist of an orderly set of questions moving from the head and neck downward. A good model of a systemic inquiry is as follows:

1. General
   - How have you been feeling?
   - Have you had any recent weight loss or weight gain?
   - Have you been feeling tired lately?
2. Head, eyes, ears, nose, throat

   Head
   - Have you ever had any problems with or injuries to your head?
   - Have you had any headaches?
   - Have you experienced any dizziness or lightheadedness?

   Eyes
   - Have you ever had any problems with your vision?
   - Have you noticed any changes in your vision?
   - Have you noticed any blurred vision or double vision?
   - Have you noticed any pain or redness of your eyes?
   - Have you noticed any spots or flecks in your visual fields?

   Ears
   - Have you ever had any problems with your ears?
   - Have you experienced any changes in your hearing?
   - Have you noticed any drainage from your ears?
   - Have you ever experienced any ringing in your ears?
   - Have you ever had any difficulty with your balance?

Nose
- Have you ever had any problems with your nose?
- Have you had any drainage from your nose?
- Do you have any problems or pain from your sinuses?
- Do you ever have any nosebleeds?
- Do you have any nasal drainage dripping down into your throat?

Throat
- Have you ever had any problems with your throat?
- Have you had any sore throats?
- Do you ever experience bleeding gums?
- When was your last visit to your dentist?
- Do you have artificial dentition?

3. Neck
- Have you ever had any problems with your neck?
- Have you ever noticed any lumps in your neck?
- Have you had any stiffness of your neck?
- Have you noticed any difficulty swallowing?

4. Cardiovascular
- Have you ever had any problems with your heart?
- Do you ever experience chest pain?
- Do you ever feel palpitations?
- Do you ever feel short of breath?
- Do you ever wake up during the night feeling short of breath?
- Do you ever notice any swelling of your legs?

5. Respiratory
- Have you ever had any problems with your breathing?
- Are you ever short of breath? If so, when?
- Do you have a cough? If so, is the cough productive?
- Do you ever have any chest pain?

6. Breast
   - Have you ever had any problems with your breasts?
   - Do you do self-breast examinations? How often?
   - Do you ever have painful breasts?
   - Have you ever noticed any lumps?
   - Do you have any nipple discharge?

7. Gastrointestinal
   - Have you ever had any problems with your stomach or bowels?
   - How is your appetite?
   - Have you noticed any change in your appetite?
   - Do you have any difficulty swallowing?
   - Do you ever experience heartburn?
   - Do you ever experience abdominal pain?
   - Have you ever vomited blood?
   - Are your bowel movements regular?
   - Have you ever noticed any blood in your stool?

8. Urinary
   - Have you ever had any problems with urination?
   - Do you have any pain during urination?
   - Do you notice any increased frequency of urination?
   - Do you have any blood in your urine?
   - Male

     Is your urinary stream normal?
     Do you notice any reduced force of the urinary stream?
     Do you ever have any difficulty urinating (hesitancy)?
     Do you ever have any dribbling (incontinence)?

9. Musculoskeletal
   - Have you ever had any problems with your bones or joints?
   - Do you have any joint stiffness?
   - Do you ever have any pain, swelling, or redness of any joints?
   - Do you have any limitation of activity due to muscle or joint pain?

10. Neurological
    - Have you ever had any neurologic problems?
    - Do you ever experience dizziness?
    - Have you ever fainted?
    - Have you ever experienced any numbness or paralysis? If so, where?
    - Do you have any weakness of your arms or legs?

11. Hematologic
    - Have you ever had any bleeding problems?
    - Do you ever experience easy bruising?
    - Have you ever had a blood transfusion for any reason?

12. Psychiatric
    - Have you ever had any psychiatric illnesses?
    - Have you ever had any problems with depression?
    - Have you ever had any problems with anxiety?
    - Have you ever had any suicidal thoughts (if yes to any of the above)?

COMPONENTS OF A COMPLETE PHYSICAL EXAMINATION

General Assessment

Observe the patient as he/she enters the room. Observe the patient's gait, height, sexual development, and posture. Observe the patient's clothing and hygiene. Be aware of any odors on the patient's breath or body.

Vital Signs

As the name indicates, these are vital components of any examination.

- Temperature
- Pulse
- Rate
- Rhythm
- Volume
- Character
- Condition of the vessel wall
- Comparison of both radial arteries
- Assess for radio-femoral delay
- Blood pressure

    Measure in three positions

    Sitting

    Standing

    Supine

    Measure the blood pressure by palpation of the radial artery in any new patient before auscultation over the brachial artery.

    Compare the blood pressure in both arms in one of the three positions.

▦ Respirations
    Rate
    Rhythm
    Regularity
    Thoracic (female) or abdominal (male)

Skin

▦ When examining any mucosal surface or any area of potentially infected or broken skin *remember to use gloves*
▦ Inspect for lesions, scars, and rashes
▦ Inspect the nails and the hair

Head and Neck

▦ Examine and palpate the head
    Size, shape, contour, deformities, suture lines
    Facial expression and symmetry
    Abnormal movements of the face
▦ Examine the scalp
    Hair distribution and texture
    Swellings
    Nits and lice
▦ Examine the oral cavity (have patient remove artificial dentition, if necessary)
    Lips
    Buccal mucosa
    Gums and teeth
    Roof of the mouth
    Hard palate
    Soft palate
    Uvula

Pharynx

Tonsils

Tongue

Floor of the mouth

Salivary glands

Wharton's ducts

Stensen's ducts

▪ Examine and palpate the neck

Anatomical land marks

Lymph nodes

Position of the trachea

▪ Thyroid gland (isthmus and lateral lobes)

Inspect (directly and on swallowing)

Palpate (directly and on swallowing)

Auscultate

Ears, Nose, and Sinuses

Ears

▪ Inspect the external ears for deformities, discharge, symmetry, lesions, inflammation

▪ Palpate

Tragus

Auricle

Mastoid process

▪ Inspect the external canal with an ear speculum (use the largest speculum that the ear canal can accommodate)

▪ Inspect the tympanic membrane for color, cone of light, handle of malleus, incus, perforations, and retractions

▪ Perform the whisper test

▪ Perform Weber's test

▪ Perform Rinne's test

Nose and sinuses

- Inspect the nostrils for patency, asymmetry, deformities, color, and discharge
- Inspect the nasal mucosa bilaterally, using the nasal speculum, for color, discharge, bleeding, and nasal polyps
- Inspect the nasal septum for deviation or perforation
- Palpate the frontal and maxillary sinuses
- Transilluminate the frontal and the maxillary sinuses (remember this should be done in a darkened room)

Eyes

- Examine the eyebrows for hair distribution and rashes
- Examine the eyes for alignment
- Examine the eye lids for swellings, lesions, ptosis, or lid retraction
- Check the visual acuity and the peripheral visual fields with and without any corrective lenses used by the patient
- Examine the conjunctiva for color, inflammation, or lesions
- Examine the lacrimal punctae and lacrimal sac for obstruction, discharge, or inflammation
- Examine the anterior chamber for clarity. Note any abnormal contents (e.g., blood, pus)
- Examine the extraocular muscles (H-test, cover/uncover, corneal reflection, and accommodation)
- Examine the iris for color, inflammation, arcus, or other abnormalities
- Note any surgical scars
- Examine the pupils for equality, shape, lens opacities, and reflexes (direct and consensual)
- Using the opthalmoscope, observe the retina (remember this should be done in a darkened room)

Cardiovascular System

- Examine the face for pallor or cyanosis
- Examine the hands for clubbing, cyanosis, or signs of bacterial endocarditis (Janeway lesions, Osler's nodes, and splinter hemorrhages)
- Examine the lower extremities bilaterally for pitting edema (dorsum of the foot, posterior medial malleolus, and anterior tibia)
- Examine the neck

  Examine the jugular venous pulse wave pattern

  Measure the jugular venous pressure and assess for any sustained hepato-jugular reflux

  Assess the carotid arteries for bruits

- Inspect the precordium for shape, symmetry, apical beat, and pulsations
- Note any surgical scars
- Palpate for tenderness
- Palpate the cardiac areas as follows:

  Aortic

  Pulmonic

  Erb's point

  Tricuspid

  Mitral

- Locate the apex and note the site, size, and character of the apical beat
- Palpate for pulsations and thrills in other cardiac areas including the epigastrium
- Look for a right ventricular heave
- Percuss the right and left borders of the heart
- Auscultate all areas with both the bell and the diaphragm (remember to auscultate in the special positions: left lateral recumbent and aortic)

Respiratory System

- Examine the head, neck, and chest for the use of accessory muscles of respiration
- Examine the hands and the face for cyanosis and for the presence of finger clubbing
- Listen for hoarseness of the voice, wheezing, and coughing
- Inspect the nose for lesions
- Examine the throat for lesions
- Palpate the trachea for deviation
- Examine the neck for lymphadenopathy
- Inspect the anterior chest for symmetry and deformities
- Palpate the chest for tenderness, tactile vocal fremitus, and chest excursion
- Percuss symmetrical areas of the chest starting from the apex
- Auscultate starting from the apices (during percussion and auscultation always compare the same areas on each side)
- Assess the character of the breath sounds
- Assess vocal resonance
- Assess for egophony
- Assess for whispering pectoriloquy
- Repeat all examinations on the posterior chest
- Assess the level of the diaphragm on the posterior chest by palpation and percussion

Abdomen

- Examine the mouth for signs of vitamin deficiencies (angular cheilitis, smooth bald tongue, etc.)
- Examine the mouth for presence and status of teeth and the presence of any dental caries
- Examine the hands and the arms for signs of hepatic failure (palmar erythema, leukonychia, asterixis)

- Examine the conjunctiva and the mucous membranes for signs of jaundice
- Examine the anterior chest for spider angiomas and gynecomastia
- Expose the abdomen from the mid chest to the thighs
- Inspect the abdomen for shape, size, color, symmetry, striae, hair distribution, scars, dilated venous patterns (caput medusae or obstruction of the inferior vena cava), visible peristalsis, visible pulsations and fetal movements (if relevant)
- Auscultate the abdomen for bowel sounds, bruits over the renal arteries, and friction rubs over the spleen and the liver
- Palpate the abdomen starting away from any area of pain or tenderness

    Light palpation

    Deep palpation (check for any masses or areas of tenderness)

    Assess the lower border of the liver

    Assess the tip of the spleen (patient lying flat and also on his/her right side)

    Palpate the kidneys

    Percuss the upper and the lower borders of the liver, the spleen, and the bladder

- Evaluate for a fluid wave and shifting dullness
- If appendicitis is suspected, check for

    Rebound tenderness

    Rovsing sign

    Psoas sign

    Obturator sign

- If cholecystitis is suspected, check for

    Murphy's sign

    Boas' sign

- In any patient in whom you suspect significant abdominal pathology do a digital rectal examination (in the CSE, state to the patient that you wish to do this but will not do so during this examination)

Musculoskeletal System

- Examine individual groups of joints
- Compare symmetrical joints
- Inspect each joint for swelling, redness, deformities, condition of the surrounding tissues, and active range of motion
- Palpate each joint for tenderness, warmth, and crepitus. If the active range of motion is impaired, check the passive range of motion
- Examine the axial skeleton (temporomandibular joints, cervical, thoracic, and lumbar spine) in the same manner
- Perform additional tests for the knee joint

    Bulge sign

    Ballottement

    Drawer sign and assessment of collateral ligaments

    McMurray's test

- Examine for sciatic nerve compression—straight leg raising test
- Examine for hip flexion contractures—Thomas' test
- Examine for median nerve compression—Phalen's test and Tinel's sign

Peripheral Vascular System

- Inspect the upper and lower extremities for size and symmetry
- Examine the nails, hair, and skin
- Observe any ulcers or gangrene (always remember to inspect the soles of the feet, especially in diabetic patients)
- Palpate temperature in both the upper and the lower extremities, comparing both limbs (remember to use the backs of your hands for this)
- Palpate pulses

    Dorsalis pedis

    Posterior tibial

    Popliteal

      Femoral

      Radial

      Ulnar

      Brachial

- Perform Allen's test
- Perform Buerger's test
- If you suspect that the patient has venous problems, assess for edema and measure the size of the calf. Perform the Trendelenberg test, the manual compression test, the Pratt's test, and the Homan's test

Central Nervous System

- Evaluate mental status (a mini-mental state examination can be used)

      Orientation to person, place, and time

      Level of consciousness

      Short-term memory

      Long-term memory

      Abstract or concrete thinking

- Observe the patient's gait and speech
- Examine all cranial nerves (I–XII)

      CN I

         Test nostrils for patency

         Ask the patient to identify common aromatic (nonirritant) substances

      CN II

         Test visual acuity

         Test pupillary reflexes (direct and consensual)

         Test accommodation reflexes

      CN III, IV, VI

         Assess pupillary reactions to light

         Assess corneal reflection

         Perform H-test for extraocular muscles

CN V

   Assess pain, crude touch, and fine touch in each division of the nerve

   Elicit corneal reflex

   Assess strength of muscles of mastication

   Assess the jaw jerk

CN VII

   Ask patient to wrinkle forehead, close eyes, smile, and blow out cheeks

CN VIII

   Perform whisper, Weber, and Rinne tests

CN IX, X

   Assess movements of the soft palate

   Assess gag reflex

CN XI

   Assess strength of trapezius and sternocleidomastoid muscles

CN XII

   Ask patient to protrude tongue (assess for fasciculations, atrophy, and
      deviations)

Sensory System

- Check for pain, crude touch, and fine touch in all parts of the body
- Check sensations carried by the dorsal columns

   Romberg's test

   Proprioception at fingers and toes

   Vibratory sense

- Check sensations of the parietal cortex

   Stereognosis

   Graphesthesia

   2-point discrimination

   Point localization

   Extinction

Motor System

▪ Inspect the motor system for atrophy, fasciculations, and involuntary movements

▪ Palpate all limbs for muscle tone

▪ Check all major muscle groups for power

Remember muscle strength is graded on a scale of 0–5

0 — No contraction

1 — Small amount of contraction

2 — Active movement (without gravity)

3 — Active movement (against gravity)

4 — Active movement against some resistance

5 — Active movement against full resistance

▪ Check all reflexes

Remember reflexes are graded on a scale of 0–4

0 — No reflex present

1 — Slightly decreased

2 — Normal

3 — Slightly increased

4 — Markedly increased, brisk

Abdominal

Plantar

Biceps

Triceps

Brachioradialis

Knee

Ankle

Cerebellum

- Ask the patient to walk in a straight line, heel to toe
- Ask the patient to walk in a straight line on his/her heels
- Ask the patient to walk in a straight line on his/her toes
- Ask the patient to perform the finger–nose test
- Ask the patient to perform the knee–heel–shin test
- Check for dysdiadochokinesia (in both hands and feet)

COMPLETE WRITE-UP

Remember: The write-up should be legible. No points will be given if the examiners are unable to read what you have written.

Areas which will be evaluated include the following:

1. *Organization*—Is the write-up easy to interpret? Does the content flow smoothly from one area to the next?
2. *Accuracy*—Does the write-up reflect the data obtained during the patient encounter? Is the write-up complete?
3. *Analysis*—Is the differential diagnosis appropriate? Is there information elsewhere in the write-up to support each differential diagnosis?
4. *Management*—Is the follow-up appropriate? Does the follow-up correspond to the differential diagnoses listed?
5. *Clarity*—Is the note legible? Is the use of language appropriate?

Example: Ectopic Pregnancy

Chief Complaint

▧ Abdominal pain for the past 24 hours.

History of Presenting Illness

The patient is a 23-year-old female complaining of abdominal pain for the past 24 hours. She describes the pain as dull and aching and located in the pelvic area. The pain does not radiate. The patient rates the pain a 7 on a scale of 1–10, with 10 being the worst. The pain has been worsening over the 24 hours since the onset. She has had no nausea, vomiting, or diarrhea. Patient denies fever. Her last menstrual period was approximately 5 weeks ago. Patient reports that her periods are often irregular but never as late as this. She is sexually active with one partner, her husband, and denies vaginal discharge. She and her husband use condoms as a method of birth control. She has no dysuria/frequency or urgency. The patient has been healthy in the past and denies ever having experienced this pain before. Her appetite has been poor since the onset of the pain. She has not taken any medications to try to relieve the pain. The patient denies constipation and reports that her last bowel movement was 1 day ago.

Medical History

▩ Urinary tract infection, 1 year ago

Surgical History

▩ Tonsillectomy, age 6

Medications

▩ Tylenol as needed

Social History

▩ Patient lives with her husband and their 2-year-old child (female). Both are in good health
▩ There are no pets at home
▩ The patient is employed as a bank teller
▩ She smokes approximately half a pack of cigarettes per day
▩ She denies the use of alcohol

Family History

▩ Patient's mother and father are alive
▩ Her mother and her maternal grandmother suffer from hypertension
▩ Her maternal grandfather suffered from asthma
▩ She has three male siblings who are all healthy

Obstetric/Gynecologic History

▩ Menstrual periods approximately every 28 days
▩ She has no dysmenorrhea, menorrhagia or metrorrhagia

▪ She has had one pregnancy 2 years ago, resulting in the vaginal delivery of a healthy female infant
▪ Her last menstrual period was approximately 5 weeks ago
▪ Her last pap smear was 9 months ago. She has no history of abnormal pap smears
▪ She is sexually active with one partner and they use condoms
▪ She has no history of sexually transmitted diseases

Physical Examination (Focused Examination)

▪ General: 23-year-old Caucasian female in mild distress
▪ Vitals

Temperature: 98.1°F

Pulse: 94/minute

Blood pressure: 134/86 mm Hg

Respirations: 14/minute

▪ Eyes: No conjunctival pallor noted
▪ Mouth

No cracks/fissures noted

Mucous membranes moist

No pallor

No dental caries noted

▪ Abdomen

No ecchymosis visible

No visible masses

No striae noted

No visible peristalsis

Bowel sounds present in all quadrants

No bruits heard

No friction rubs over the spleen or liver

Mild tenderness in the left lower quadrant to light palpation

Marked tenderness in the left lower quadrant to deep palpation

No hepatosplenomegaly
No costovertebral angle (CVA) tenderness
No shifting dullness
No referred rebound tenderness
No rebound tenderness
Rovsing sign negative
Psoas sign negative
Obturator sign negative

Differential Diagnosis

1. Ectopic pregnancy
2. Ruptured ovarian cyst
3. Appendicitis
4. Ovarian torsion
5. Urinary tract infection

Follow-Up

1. Digital rectal examination (DRE)
2. Beta human chorionic gonadotrophin (β-HCG)
3. Urinalysis (U/A)
4. Complete blood count (CBC)
5. Abdominal ultrasound

ACCEPTABLE ABBREVIATIONS

Note: This is not a complete list of acceptable abbreviations that may be used during the examination but rather a representative sample of common abbreviations that may be used on a patient note. If you are uncertain about the correct abbreviation on exam day, write it out.

Vital Signs

BP	Blood pressure
HR	Heart rate
R	Respirations
T	Temperature

Laboratory Tests and Follow-Up

ABG	Arterial blood gas
β-HCG	Beta human chorionic gonadotrophin
BUN	Blood urea nitrogen
CABG	Coronary artery bypass grafting
CBC	Complete blood count
CK level	Creatine phosphokinase level
CK-MB	Creatine kinase (myocardial component)
CPR	Cardiopulmonary resuscitation
CT	Computerized tomography
CVP	Central venous pressure
CXR	Chest X-ray
DRE	Digital rectal examination
ECG	Electrocardiogram
EcHO	Echocardiogram
EEG	Electroencephalogram
EGD	Esophagogastroduodenoscopy

EMG	Electromyography
ERCP	Endoscopic retrograde cholangiopancreatography
ESR	Erythrocyte sedimentation rate
Free T3	Free triiodothyroxine
Free T4	Free thyroxine
HgA1C	Glycosylated hemoglobin level
IM	Intramuscular
IV	Intravenous
LFT's	Liver function tests
LP	Lumbar puncture
MRI	Magnetic resonance imaging
PFT's	Pulmonary function tests
PPD	Purified protein derivative (tuberculin skin test)
PT	Prothrombin time
PTT	Partial prothrombin time
RBC	Red blood cells
RF	Rheumatoid factor
TPA	Tissue plasminogen activator
TSH	Thyroid stimulating hormone
U/A	Urinalysis
VDRL	Venereal Disease Research Laboratory
WBC	White blood cells

Units of Measure

C	Centigrade
cm	Centimeter
F	Fahrenheit
g	Gram
hr	Hour
kg	Kilogram
m	Meter
μg	Microgram
mg	Miligram
min	Minute
oz	Ounces
lbs	Pounds

Other

ABD	Abdomen
AIDS	Acquired immune deficiency syndrome
AP	Anteroposterior
CCU	Cardiac care unit
CHF	Congestive heart failure
COPD	Chronic obstructive pulmonary disease
CVA	Cerebrovascular accident
DM	Diabetes mellitus
DTR	Deep tendon reflexes
ED	Emergency department
EMT	Emergency medical technician
ENT	Ear, nose, and throat
EOM	Extraocular muscles
ETOH	Alcohol
Ext	Extremities
FH	Family history
GI	Gastrointestinal
GU	Genitourinary
HEENT	Head, ears, eyes, nose, and throat
HIV	Human immunodeficiency virus
HTN	Hypertension
JVD	Jugular venous distention
JVP	Jugular venous pulse or pressure
KUB	Kidney, ureter, and bladder
LMP	Last menstrual period
MI	Myocardial infarction
MVA	Motor vehicle accident
Neuro	Neurologic
NIDDM	Non-insulin-dependent diabetes mellitus
NKA	No known allergies
NKDA	No known drug allergies
NL	Normal limits
NSAID	Nonsteroidal anti-inflammatory drug
NSR	Normal sinus rhythm

PA	Posteroanterior
PERRLA	Pupils equal, round, reactive to light and accomodation
Po	Per os (orally)
TIA	Transient ischemic attack
URI	Upper respiratory infection
WNL	Within normal limits
Yo	Year old

SECTION II

Clinical Cases and Checklists

CASE 1

A 65-year-old female is brought to the emergency department by her husband. He noticed that she seems to be having some difficulty with her speech and some confusion.

The patient's husband reports that approximately 4 hours ago he noticed that his wife had developed some difficulty with her speech. She seemed to be confusing object's names. About 1 month ago she had an episode where she complained that she could not open her left eye, but this lasted only a few seconds. She now gives a clear history with normal speech. Her medical history is significant for hypertension and two previous heart attacks. She has not experienced chest pain with this episode. She used to smoke cigarettes, about a pack per day, but gave up smoking 3 years ago at the time of her first heart attack. She lives at home with her husband.

Patient History Checklist

☐ Patient's name
☐ Patient's age
☐ Patient's address
☐ Patient's occupation
☐ Patient's presenting complaint
☐ Time of onset of symptoms
☐ Previous episode of symptoms
☐ Presence of aphasia
☐ Presence of ataxia
☐ Presence of numbness
☐ Presence of loss of motor function
☐ Episodes of impaired vision
☐ History of abnormal movements and/or tremors
☐ Incontinence of urine
☐ Presence of dizziness

- ☐ Presence of nausea/vomiting
- ☐ Presence of fatigue
- ☐ Presence of irritability
- ☐ Difficulty concentrating
- ☐ Difficulty sleeping
- ☐ Presence of chest pain
- ☐ Presence of shortness of breath
- ☐ Risk factors
  - ☐ Hypertension
  - ☐ Heart disease
  - ☐ Diabetes mellitus
  - ☐ History of transient ischemic attacks
  - ☐ Cigarette smoking
- ☐ History of trauma
- ☐ Medical history
- ☐ Hospital admissions
- ☐ Surgical history
- ☐ Medications, including over-the-counter medications, prescription medications, and illicit drugs

Differential Diagnosis

1. _____   6. _____
2. _____   7. _____
3. _____   8. _____
4. _____   9. _____
5. _____

Physical Examination Checklist

- ☐ Overall assessment
- ☐ Vitals
  - ☐ Temperature
  - ☐ Pulse—assess for arrhythmias
  - ☐ Blood pressure—assess for hypertension
  - ☐ Respirations

- ☐ Evaluate mental status
  - ☐ Orientation to person, place, and time
  - ☐ Level of consciousness
  - ☐ Short-term memory
  - ☐ Long-term memory
  - ☐ Observe the patient's gait and speech
- ☐ Examine the head
  - ☐ Assess for masses, ecchymosis, lacerations, tenderness
  - ☐ Examine the tongue for bite injury
- ☐ Examine the ears
  - ☐ Assess the external ear canal for fluid drainage
  - ☐ Assess the tympanic membranes
- ☐ Examine all cranial nerves (I–XII)
- ☐ Examine the sensory system
  - ☐ Check for pain and crude touch in all parts of the body
  - ☐ Romberg's test
  - ☐ Proprioception at fingers and toes
  - ☐ Vibratory sense
  - ☐ Stereognosis
  - ☐ Graphesthesia
  - ☐ 2-point discrimination
  - ☐ Point localization
  - ☐ Extinction
- ☐ Examine the motor system
  - ☐ Inspect the motor system for atrophy, fasciculations, and involuntary movements
  - ☐ Palpate all limbs for muscle tone
  - ☐ Check all major muscle groups for power
  - ☐ Check all reflexes
    - ☐ Abdominal
    - ☐ Plantar
    - ☐ Biceps
    - ☐ Triceps
    - ☐ Brachioradialis
    - ☐ Knee
    - ☐ Ankle

☐ Examine the cerebellum
  ☐ Ask the patient to walk in a straight line, heel to toes
  ☐ Ask the patient to walk in a straight line on his/her heels
  ☐ Ask the patient to walk in a straight line on his/her toes
  ☐ Ask the patient to perform the finger–nose test
  ☐ Ask the patient to perform the knee–heel–shin test
  ☐ Check for dysdiadochokinesia

Physical Examination Findings

General: 65-year-old female, no acute distress
Vitals:

Pulse — 88/minute	Temperature — 97.8°F
BP — 144/64 mm Hg	Respirations — 16/minute

Mental status:

Patient oriented to person, place, and time

Patient awake and alert

Long-term memory intact

Short-term memory intact

No abnormal gait observed

Speech appropriate

HEENT:

Head — No masses, ecchymosis, lacerations, or tenderness appreciated

  No bite injury to tongue

Ears — No drainage noted

  Tympanic membranes visualized bilaterally

Cranial nerves: I–XII intact

Sensory system: Sensation intact bilaterally

Motor system:

No atrophy noted

No fasciculations

Normal muscle tone noted in all extremities

Normal power observed in all extremities
Deep tendon reflexes intact
Abdominal reflex present
Plantar reflex down going
Cerebellum: No abnormalities noted

Differential Diagnosis

1. _____   3. _____
2. _____   4. _____

Follow-Up

1. _____   4. _____
2. _____   5. _____
3. _____

See Section III for differential diagnosis, appropriate follow-up, and brief case review.

A 43-year-old female is brought to the outpatient department by her husband. He reports that her behavior has been strange over the past 2 weeks.

He has noticed that his wife seems to be "acting funny." She seems to be having difficulty concentrating for any significant period of time. She also seems to be unable to sit still and is constantly fidgeting and finding things to do. He does not think that his wife has been sleeping through the night as there have been multiple times over the past 2 weeks that he has woken up and she has not been in the bed. He has noticed that she seems to be dressing differently from her usual. He finds that her dress is flamboyant and she is applying much more makeup than she usually does. When his wife is asked how she is feeling she replies that she has never felt better and does not know what her husband is talking about. She does not seem to be interested in the care of their two children at the moment and has been occasionally forgetting to feed them. She has never had an episode like this in the past. She does have episodes of depression. When she is in one of her "depressed moods" she becomes very tearful, tired, and tends to sleep a lot.

Patient History Checklist

- ☐ Patient's name
- ☐ Patient's age
- ☐ Patient's address
- ☐ Patient's occupation
- ☐ Patient's presenting complaint
- ☐ Duration of symptoms
- ☐ Presence of stress
- ☐ Presence of hallucinations
- ☐ Presence of delusions
- ☐ Presence of irritability
- ☐ Presence of restlessness

- ☐ Difficulty concentrating
- ☐ Difficulty sleeping
- ☐ Increased sexual drive
- ☐ Changes in appetite
- ☐ Presence of weight loss/gain
- ☐ Amount of weight loss/weight gain
- ☐ Time period of weight loss/weight gain
- ☐ Medical history
- ☐ Hospital admissions
- ☐ Surgical history
- ☐ Medications
- ☐ Social history
    - ☐ Smoking (how much?)
    - ☐ Alcohol (how much?)
    - ☐ Drug use (Specific drugs, including method of use)
    - ☐ Family situation
    - ☐ Work situation
    - ☐ Ability to function at work
    - ☐ Ability to function at home
    - ☐ Presence of support system
- ☐ Suicidal ideation
    - ☐ Suicide plan
    - ☐ Previous suicide attempts
- ☐ Homicidal ideation
- ☐ Family history
    - ☐ Bipolar disorder
    - ☐ Psychiatric illnesses
    - ☐ Drug abuse
    - ☐ Depression
    - ☐ Heart disease
    - ☐ Diabetes
    - ☐ Thyroid disease
    - ☐ Cancer
    - ☐ Others

Differential Diagnosis

1. _____   6. _____
2. _____   7. _____
3. _____   8. _____
4. _____   9. _____
5. _____

Physical Examination Checklist

☐ Evaluate mental status
  ☐ Orientation to person, place, and time
  ☐ Level of consciousness
  ☐ Short-term memory
  ☐ Long-term memory
  ☐ Abstract or concrete thinking
  ☐ Mood and affect
☐ Observe the patient's gait and speech
☐ Perform a complete physical examination if time permits

Physical Examination Findings

General: 43-year-old female, no acute distress. Patient restless during interview. Unable to maintain eye contact. Difficult to engage in conversation.

Vitals:

Pulse—88/minute   Temperature—99.1°F
BP—142/90 mm Hg   Respirations—16/minute

Mental status:

Patient oriented to person, place, and time

Patient awake and alert

Long-term memory intact

Short-term memory impaired

No abnormal gait observed

Speech rapid but appropriate

Differential Diagnosis

1. _____   3. _____
2. _____   4. _____

Follow-Up

1. _____   4. _____
2. _____   5. _____
3. _____

See Section III for differential diagnosis, appropriate follow-up, and brief case review.

CASE 3

A 32-year-old female is seen in the outpatient department complaining of difficulty swallowing.

The patient reports that she has been having some difficulty swallowing for the past 3 months. The problem seems to be worsening. She complains that it is difficult to swallow both liquids and solids. She finds that sometimes after taking a bite of food she has a choking/coughing episode and feels that it is difficult to breath. She has never experienced similar symptoms. She has no other complaints. She states that her appetite has been poor; however, she has not noticed any weight loss. She denies nausea or vomiting and has been afebrile since the onset of the symptoms. She complains that she often experiences chest pain following eating. She describes the pain as centrally located in her chest and as a burning sensation. She does not take any medications. She drinks approximately 2 glasses of wine per day and smokes approximately 15 cigarettes per day.

Patient History Checklist

- ☐ Patient's name
- ☐ Patient's age
- ☐ Patient's address
- ☐ Patient's occupation
- ☐ Patient's presenting complaint
- ☐ Presence of difficulty swallowing
- ☐ Presence of difficulty swallowing solid foods
- ☐ Presence of difficulty swallowing liquids
- ☐ Duration of symptoms
- ☐ Presence of chest pain
- ☐ History of the pain
  - ☐ Site
  - ☐ Onset

- ☐ Duration
- ☐ Intensity
- ☐ Radiation
- ☐ Character
- ☐ Exacerbating factors
- ☐ Relieving factors
- ☐ Medications used to try to relieve the pain
- ☐ Changes in weight (loss/gain)
- ☐ Amount of weight loss/weight gain
- ☐ Time period of weight loss/weight gain
- ☐ Changes in bowel movements
- ☐ Changes in appetite (increased/decreased)
- ☐ Presence of melena
- ☐ Presence of hematemesis
- ☐ Presence of nausea/vomiting
- ☐ Presence of cough
- ☐ Presence of shortness of breath
- ☐ Presence of fever
- ☐ Presence of swelling in the neck
- ☐ History of travel/residence abroad (especially to/in South America)
- ☐ History of psychiatric illness
- ☐ Medical history
- ☐ Hospital admissions
- ☐ Surgical history
- ☐ Medications
- ☐ Family history
  - ☐ Thyroid disease
  - ☐ Gastric ulcers
  - ☐ Heart disease
  - ☐ Diabetes
  - ☐ Cancer
  - ☐ Psychiatric illnesses
  - ☐ Others
- ☐ Social history
  - ☐ Smoking
  - ☐ Alcohol
  - ☐ Other drug use

Differential Diagnosis

1. _____   6. _____
2. _____   7. _____
3. _____   8. _____
4. _____   9. _____
5. _____

Physical Examination Checklist

- ☐ Overall assessment
- ☐ Vitals
  - ☐ Temperature
  - ☐ Pulse
  - ☐ Blood pressure
  - ☐ Respirations
- ☐ Examine the neck
  - ☐ Assess for any swellings
  - ☐ Assess for normal thyroid gland
- ☐ Examine the abdomen
  - ☐ Inspect
  - ☐ Auscultate
  - ☐ Light palpation
  - ☐ Deep palpation
  - ☐ Assess for organomegaly (palpation and percussion)
  - ☐ Assess for muscular rigidity
  - ☐ Assess for rebound tenderness
- ☐ Cardiovascular system
  - ☐ Inspect the precordium
  - ☐ Shape
  - ☐ Scars
  - ☐ Pulses
  - ☐ Apex
- ☐ Palpate the precordium
  - ☐ Tenderness
  - ☐ Pulses
  - ☐ Apex

☐ Thrills
☐ Heaves
☐ Percuss the heart borders
☐ Auscultate with the bell
   ☐ Aortic area
   ☐ Pulmonic area
   ☐ Erb's point
   ☐ Tricuspid area
   ☐ Apex (mitral) area
☐ Auscultate with the diaphragm
   ☐ Aortic area
   ☐ Pulmonic area
   ☐ Erb's point
   ☐ Tricuspid area
   ☐ Apex (mitral) area
☐ Auscultate with the bell—patient in left lateral recumbent position
☐ Auscultate with the diaphragm—patient in aortic position
☐ Respiratory system—examine the thorax
   ☐ Inspect
      ☐ Size
      ☐ Shape
      ☐ Symmetry
      ☐ Movement
      ☐ Deformities of the ribs
      ☐ Deformities of the spine
      ☐ Scars
   ☐ Palpate
      ☐ Tenderness
      ☐ Excursion
      ☐ Tactile fremitus
      ☐ Chest dimensions
      ☐ Position of the diaphragm
   ☐ Percuss
      ☐ All areas comparing side to side
      ☐ Diaphragm excursion (left)
      ☐ Diaphragm excursion (right)
   ☐ Auscultate
      ☐ All areas comparing side to side

   ☐ Breath sounds
   ☐ Vocal resonance
   ☐ Whispering pectoriloquy
   ☐ Aegophony
☐ Indicate to the patient that you would like to perform a digital rectal examination but will not do so during this examination

Physical Examination Findings

General: 32-year-old female, no acute distress
Vitals:

Pulse—74/minute	Temperature—97.9°F
BP—114/74 mm Hg	Respirations—14/minute

Neck:

No swellings noted

Trachea midline

No goiter appreciated

No thyroid nodules appreciated

Abdomen:

No ecchymosis visible

No visible masses

No striae noted

No visible peristalsis

Bowel sounds present in all quadrants

No bruits heard

No friction rubs over the spleen or liver

No tenderness to palpation

No hepatosplenomegaly

No rebound tenderness noted

Cardiovascular system:

Precordium normal shape and size

No abnormal pulsations appreciated

Apical, suprasternal, and abdominal pulsations observed

No tenderness to palpation

Apical, suprasternal, and abdominal pulsations all palpable

No thrills or heaves

S1, S2 heard, no murmurs

Respiratory system:

Thorax normal size and shape

No asymmetry noted

No scars or deformities noted

No tenderness to palpation

Excursion equal bilaterally

Tactile fremitus equal bilaterally

No increased anteroposterior diameter

Resonant to percussion bilaterally

Level of the diaphragms equal bilaterally

Breath sounds appreciated throughout

No wheezing noted

No whispering pectoriloquy noted

No aegophony noted

Differential Diagnosis

1. _____   3. _____
2. _____   4. _____

Follow-Up

1. _____   4. _____
2. _____   5. _____
3. _____

See Section III for differential diagnosis, appropriate follow-up, and brief case review.

CASE 4

A 77-year-old female complaining of hip pain.

The patient was brought to the clinic by the staff of her assisted living home. The staff at the home found the patient lying on the floor of her bathroom. The patient was confused upon being found and could not give any information as to how or at what time the fall had taken place. While transferring the patient to the clinic, a large ecchymosis was noted on her left buttock and her left posterior thigh. She complained of feeling some pain around her left buttock and was unable to weight bear at all on the left side. Her medical history is significant for hypertension, diabetes, osteoporosis, and mild congestive heart failure. She takes a variety of medications for these conditions. She has smoked cigarettes for the past 60 years, approximately 1 pack per day. She denies the use of alcohol. Her meals are provided by the home where she resides and the staff report that her appetite is fairly good and she eats a wide variety of foods.

Patient History Checklist

☐ Patient's name
☐ Patient's age
☐ Patient's address
☐ Patient's presenting complaint
☐ Absence/presence of pain
☐ History of the pain
   ☐ Site
   ☐ Onset
   ☐ Duration
   ☐ Intensity
   ☐ Radiation
   ☐ Character
   ☐ Exacerbating factors
   ☐ Relieving factors
   ☐ Medications used to relieve symptoms

- ☐ History of fall/injury
- ☐ Time of fall/injury
- ☐ Loss of consciousness at time of fall
- ☐ Presence of dizziness at time of fall
- ☐ Previous falls
- ☐ Previous fractures
- ☐ Difficulty with vision
- ☐ Presence of pain on movement
- ☐ Swelling of the affected area
- ☐ Redness of the affected area
- ☐ Presence of ecchymosis
- ☐ Presence of nausea/vomiting
- ☐ Presence of fatigue
- ☐ Medical history
- ☐ Hospital admissions
- ☐ Surgical history
- ☐ Medications (including vitamin supplements)
- ☐ Age of menopause
- ☐ Number of children
- ☐ Family history
  - ☐ Heart disease
  - ☐ Diabetes
  - ☐ Thyroid disease
  - ☐ Cancer
  - ☐ Others
- ☐ Social history
  - ☐ Smoking
  - ☐ Alcohol
  - ☐ Other drug use

Differential Diagnosis

1. _____   6. _____
2. _____   7. _____
3. _____   8. _____
4. _____   9. _____
5. _____

Physical Examination Checklist

- ☐ Overall assessment
- ☐ Vitals
    - ☐ Temperature
    - ☐ Pulse—assess for bradycardia
    - ☐ Blood pressure—assess for hypotension
    - ☐ Respirations
- ☐ Examine the extremities (bilaterally)
    - ☐ Inspect upper extremities
        - ☐ Symmetry
        - ☐ Deformities
        - ☐ Swellings
        - ☐ Areas of erythema and/or ecchymosis
    - ☐ Palpate upper extremities
        - ☐ Temperature
        - ☐ Comparing both limbs
        - ☐ Tenderness
        - ☐ Masses
    - ☐ Inspect lower extremities
        - ☐ Symmetry
        - ☐ Deformities
        - ☐ Swellings
        - ☐ Areas of erythema and/or ecchymosis
    - ☐ Palpate lower extremities
        - ☐ Temperature
        - ☐ Comparing both limbs
        - ☐ Tenderness
        - ☐ Masses
- ☐ Assess mobility of hip joints
- ☐ Assess mobility of knee joints
- ☐ Assess mobility of ankle joints
- ☐ Assess mobility of finger joints
- ☐ Assess mobility of foot joints
- ☐ Assess for external rotation of hip joint
- ☐ Check all reflexes
    - ☐ Abdominal
    - ☐ Plantar

- ☐ Biceps
- ☐ Triceps
- ☐ Brachioradialis
- ☐ Quadriceps
- ☐ Knee
- ☐ Ankle
- ☐ Palpate pulses
  - ☐ Dorsalis pedis
  - ☐ Posterior tibial
  - ☐ Popliteal
  - ☐ Femoral
  - ☐ Radial
  - ☐ Ulnar
  - ☐ Brachial
- ☐ If time permits, perform a full cardiovascular examination

Physical Examination Findings

General: 77-year-old female, lying in bed, uncomfortable appearing

Vitals:

Pulse—98/minute	Temperature—96.4°F
BP—132/68 mm Hg	Respirations—18/minute

Upper extremities:

Symmetrical

No ecchymosis, erythema, swellings, or deformities noted

No tenderness on palpation

Temperature equal bilaterally

Lower extremities:

Asymmetrical, left lower extremity appears shortened and the foot is rotated laterally

Large ecchymosis on left buttock noted

Large ecchymosis on posterior left thigh noted

No scars

Area of erythema noted over left hip region

Temperature equal bilaterally
No masses appreciated
Full active range of motion at knees, ankles, and foot joints
No active range of motion of left hip
Passive range of motion of left hip limited by pain
Deep tendon reflexes intact
Abdominal reflex present
Plantar reflex down going
All peripheral pulses palpable

Differential Diagnosis

1. _____   3. _____
2. _____   4. _____

Follow-Up

1. _____   4. _____
2. _____   5. _____
3. _____

See Section III for differential diagnosis, appropriate follow-up, and brief case review.

CASE 5

A 59-year-old female is seen in the clinic. She has been experiencing pain in her left calf while walking.

The patient has always enjoyed walking. However, since the onset of this pain she has decreased the amount of walking that she has been doing. The pain starts after walking about half a mile and she describes the pain as a dull, aching pain. She usually stops for about 5 minutes when she experiences the pain and the pain resolves. However, it comes back again after walking the same distance. Her medical history is significant for hypertension for the past 15 years. She smokes 2 packs of cigarettes a day and has done so for the past 45 years. She denies the use of alcohol.

Patient History Checklist

- ☐ Patient's name
- ☐ Patient's age
- ☐ Patient's address
- ☐ Patient's occupation
- ☐ Patient's presenting complaint
- ☐ Presence of pain
- ☐ History of the pain
    - ☐ Site
    - ☐ Onset
    - ☐ Duration
    - ☐ Intensity
    - ☐ Radiation
    - ☐ Character
    - ☐ Exacerbating factors
    - ☐ Relieving factors
- ☐ History of vascular disease
- ☐ History of diabetes

☐ History of hypertension
☐ Presence of weight loss/gain
☐ Amount of weight loss/weight gain
☐ Time period of weight loss/weight gain
☐ Medical history
☐ Hospital admissions
☐ Surgical history
☐ Medications
☐ Family history
   ☐ Heart disease
   ☐ Diabetes
   ☐ Hypertension
   ☐ Cancer
   ☐ Others
☐ Social history
   ☐ Smoking
   ☐ Alcohol
   ☐ Other drug use

Differential Diagnosis

1. _____   6. _____
2. _____   7. _____
3. _____   8. _____
4. _____   9. _____
5. _____

Physical Examination Checklist

☐ Overall assessment
☐ Vitals
   ☐ Temperature
   ☐ Pulse
   ☐ Blood pressure
   ☐ Respirations
☐ Inspect the upper and lower extremities for size and symmetry
☐ Examine the nails, hair, and skin

☐ Observe any ulcers or gangrene taking care to examine the soles of the feet
☐ Palpate temperature in both the upper and the lower extremities comparing both sides
☐ Palpate pulses
  ☐ Dorsalis pedis
  ☐ Posterior tibial
  ☐ Popliteal
  ☐ Femoral
  ☐ Radial
  ☐ Ulnar
  ☐ Brachial
☐ Perform Allen's test
☐ Perform Buerger's test
☐ Check for bruits over the abdominal aorta and both the iliofemoral arteries
☐ Examine the motor system
  ☐ Inspect the motor system for atrophy, fasciculations, and involuntary movements
  ☐ Palpate all limbs for muscle tone
  ☐ Check all major muscle groups for power
  ☐ Check all reflexes
    ☐ Abdominal
    ☐ Plantar
    ☐ Biceps
    ☐ Triceps
    ☐ Brachioradialis
    ☐ Knee
    ☐ Ankle
☐ Examine the sensory system
  ☐ Check for pain and crude touch in all parts of the body
  ☐ Romberg's test
  ☐ Proprioception at fingers and toes
  ☐ Vibratory sense
  ☐ Stereognosis
  ☐ Graphesthesia
  ☐ 2-point discrimination
  ☐ Point localization
  ☐ Extinction
☐ If time permits perform a full cardiovascular examination

Physical Examination Findings

General: 59-year-old female, no acute distress

Vitals:

    Pulse—68/minute   Temperature—98.5°F

    BP—132/92 mm Hg   Respirations—12/minute

Upper extremities:

    Symmetrical

    Temperature equal bilaterally

    No ecchymosis, erythema, swellings, or deformities noted

    No tenderness on palpation

    No ulcers or gangrene noted

    Normal hair distribution

    No thickening or ridges of the nails

Lower extremities:

    Symmetrical

    Temperature equal bilaterally

    No ecchymosis, erythema, swellings, or deformities noted

    No tenderness on palpation

    No ulcers or gangrene noted

    Normal hair distribution

    No thickening or ridges of the nails

All peripheral pulses palpable

Allen's test negative

Buerger's test negative

No bruits noted over abdominal aorta or iliofemoral arteries

Sensory system: Sensation intact bilaterally

Motor system:

    No atrophy noted

    No fasciculations

    Normal muscle tone noted in all extremities

Normal power observed in all extremities
Deep tendon reflexes intact
Sensory system: Sensation intact bilaterally

Differential Diagnosis

1. _____   3. _____
2. _____   4. _____

Follow-Up

1. _____   4. _____
2. _____   5. _____
3. _____

See Section III for differential diagnosis, appropriate follow-up, and brief case review.

CASE 6

A 65-year-old female is seen in the emergency department. She is complaining of worsening shortness of breath over the past 3 weeks.

The patient reports that she has never experienced similar symptoms in the past. She also complains of a persistent cough over the same period of time. She describes her sputum as pink and frothy. She has difficulty sleeping at night due to the shortness of breath and finds that it helps her if she sits up in the bed or sits in her recliner to sleep. Her medical history is significant for hypertension; however, she reports that she has not been to see her primary care physician for quite a few years and is not currently taking any medication for the blood pressure. She denies the use of cigarettes or alcohol.

Patient History Checklist

- ☐ Patient's name
- ☐ Patient's age
- ☐ Patient's address
- ☐ Patient's occupation
- ☐ Patient's presenting complaint
- ☐ Duration of symptoms
- ☐ Presence of cough (productive/nonproductive)
- ☐ Appearance of the sputum
- ☐ Presence of fever
- ☐ Shortness of breath
- ☐ Severity of the symptoms
- ☐ Previous episodes of symptoms
- ☐ Swelling of the extremities
- ☐ Changes in diet/salt intake
- ☐ Presence of palpitations
- ☐ Relieving factors
- ☐ Aggravating factors

☐ Medications used during this acute episode/effect of medications used
☐ Presence of chest pain
☐ Allergies
☐ Risk factors
    ☐ Family history
    ☐ Hypertension
    ☐ Diabetes
    ☐ Previous heart condition
    ☐ Smoking
    ☐ Alcohol
    ☐ Exercise
    ☐ Occupation
    ☐ Stress at present
☐ Medical history
☐ Hospital admissions
☐ Surgical history
☐ Medications

Differential Diagnosis

1. _____   6. _____
2. _____   7. _____
3. _____   8. _____
4. _____   9. _____
5. _____

Physical Examination Checklist

☐ Overall assessment
☐ Vitals
    ☐ Temperature—assess for fever
    ☐ Pulse—assess for arrhythmias
    ☐ Blood pressure—assess for hypertension
    ☐ Respirations
☐ Examine the face
    ☐ Assess mucus membranes for the presence of cyanosis or pallor

☐ Examine the extremities
    ☐ Assess for clubbing
    ☐ Assess for cyanosis
    ☐ Assess for pitting edema
☐ Examine the neck
    ☐ Examine JVP wave pattern
    ☐ Measure the JVP
    ☐ Assess hepatojugular reflux
    ☐ Carotid arteries—assess for bruits
    ☐ Assess for use of accessory muscles of respiration
    ☐ Assess the position of the trachea
☐ Respiratory system—examine the thorax
    ☐ Inspect
        ☐ Size
        ☐ Shape
        ☐ Symmetry
        ☐ Movement
        ☐ Deformities of the ribs
        ☐ Deformities of the spine
        ☐ Scars
    ☐ Palpate
        ☐ Tenderness
        ☐ Excursion
        ☐ Tactile fremitus
        ☐ Chest dimensions
        ☐ Position of the diaphragm
    ☐ Percuss
        ☐ All areas comparing side to side
        ☐ Diaphragm excursion (left)
        ☐ Diaphragm excursion (right)
    ☐ Auscultate
        ☐ All areas comparing side to side
        ☐ Breath sounds
        ☐ Adventitious sounds
        ☐ Vocal resonance
        ☐ Whispering pectoriloquy
        ☐ Aegophony

- ☐ Cardiovascular system
  - ☐ Inspect the precordium
    - ☐ Shape
    - ☐ Scars
    - ☐ Pulses
    - ☐ Apex
  - ☐ Palpate the precordium
    - ☐ Tenderness
    - ☐ Pulses
    - ☐ Apex
    - ☐ Thrills
    - ☐ Heaves
  - ☐ Percuss the heart borders
  - ☐ Auscultate with the bell
    - ☐ Aortic area
    - ☐ Pulmonic area
    - ☐ Erb's point
    - ☐ Tricuspid area
    - ☐ Apex (mitral) area
  - ☐ Auscultate with the diaphragm
    - ☐ Aortic area
    - ☐ Pulmonic area
    - ☐ Erb's point
    - ☐ Tricuspid area
    - ☐ Apex (mitral) area
  - ☐ Auscultate with the bell—patient in left lateral recumbent position
  - ☐ Auscultate with the diaphragm—patient in aortic position

Physical Examination Findings

General: 65-year-old female, mild distress
Vitals:

Pulse—98/minute   Temperature—98.9°F
BP—150/84 mm Hg   Respirations—20/minute

Mouth:

No cyanosis noted

Mucous membranes moist

No pallor

Extremities:

    No clubbing or cyanosis noted

    Moderate bilateral pitting edema of lower extremities noted

Neck:

    Increase in JVP noted

    No hepatojugular reflux noted

    No carotid bruits appreciated

    Some use of accessory muscles of respirations

    Trachea midline

Respiratory system:

    Thorax normal size and shape

    No asymmetry noted

    No scars or deformities noted

    No tenderness to palpation

    Excursion equal bilaterally

    Tactile fremitus decreased at bases bilaterally

    No increased anteroposterior diameter

    Dull to percussion at bases bilaterally

    Level of the diaphragms equal bilaterally

    Breath sounds decreased at bases bilaterally

    No wheezing noted

    Bilateral basilar crackles noted

    No whispering pectoriloquy noted

    No aegophony noted

Cardiovascular system:

    Precordium normal shape and size

    No abnormal pulsations appreciated

    Apical, suprasternal, and abdominal pulsations observed

    No tenderness to palpation

Apical, suprasternal, and abdominal pulsations all palpable
No thrills or heaves
S1, S2 heard, no murmurs

Differential Diagnosis

1. _____   3. _____
2. _____   4. _____

Follow-Up

1. _____   4. _____
2. _____   5. _____
3. _____

See Section III for differential diagnosis, appropriate follow-up, and brief case review.

CASE 7

A 32-year-old female is seen by her primary care physician complaining that she has noticed that she is having difficulty hearing.

The patient first noticed that there was a problem 2 weeks ago when she realized that she was having difficulty hearing the television when no one else seemed to be having difficulty. She denies ever having any similar problems in the past. She has not done anything unusual over the past few weeks such as swimming or diving. She does not use cotton swabs in her ears. She has not noticed any drainage from the ears. She has been afebrile and denies any pain associated with her ears. Her medical history is significant for asthma, which is well controlled with albuterol.

Patient History

- ☐ Patient's name
- ☐ Patient's age
- ☐ Patient's address
- ☐ Patient's occupation
- ☐ Patient's presenting complaint
- ☐ Duration of symptoms
- ☐ Presence of ear pain
- ☐ Presence of drainage from ears
- ☐ Presence of fever
- ☐ History of previous episodes
- ☐ Presence of ringing in the ears
- ☐ Use of cotton swabs
- ☐ Presence of dizziness
- ☐ Presence of headaches
- ☐ Presence of nausea
- ☐ Presence of vomiting
- ☐ Medical history

☐ Hospital admissions
☐ Surgical history
☐ Medications
☐ Family history
   ☐ Heart disease
   ☐ Diabetes
   ☐ Thyroid disease
   ☐ Cancer
   ☐ Others
☐ Social history
   ☐ Smoking
   ☐ Alcohol
   ☐ Other drug use

Differential Diagnosis

1. _____   6. _____
2. _____   7. _____
3. _____   8. _____
4. _____   9. _____
5. _____

Physical Examination Checklist

☐ Overall assessment
☐ Vitals
   ☐ Temperature
   ☐ Pulse
   ☐ Blood pressure
   ☐ Respirations
☐ Inspect the external ears
   ☐ Deformities
   ☐ Discharge
   ☐ Symmetry
   ☐ Lesions
   ☐ Inflammation

☐ Palpate
    ☐ Tragus
    ☐ Auricle
    ☐ Mastoid process
☐ Inspect the external canal with an ear speculum
☐ Inspect the tympanic membrane
    ☐ Color
    ☐ Cone of light
    ☐ Handle of malleus
    ☐ Incus
    ☐ Perforations
    ☐ Retractions
☐ Perform the whisper test
☐ Perform Weber's test
☐ Perform Rinne's test

Physical Examination Findings

General: 32-year-old female, no acute distress
Vitals:

    Pulse—68/minute   Temperature—98.3°F
    BP—114/76 mm Hg   Respirations—14/minute

Ears:

    Symmetrical

    No deformities, lesions, erythema, inflammation, or drainage noted

    No tenderness on palpation of the tragus, auricle, or mastoid process

    No erythema or lesions visualized in the external canal

    Excess cerumen noted in the left external ear canal

    Tympanic membranes visualized on the right, no perforations, no retractions

    Unable to visualize tympanic membrane on the left due to cerumen in the external canal

    Whisper test—decreased on left

    Weber's test lateralized to the left

    Rinne's test—bone conduction greater that air conduction on the left

Differential Diagnosis

1. _____   3. _____
2. _____   4. _____

Follow-Up

1. _____   4. _____
2. _____   5. _____
3. _____

See Section III for differential diagnosis, appropriate follow-up, and brief case review.

A 55-year-old male is seen in the emergency department complaining of severe abdominal pain which started several hours ago.

The pain is located in the middle/left upper abdominal area and radiates to his lower middle back. The patient relates the pain to eating as he had just finished a large meal before the initial onset of the pain. He describes the pain as a twisting, stabbing pain, which has been gradually worsening. He reports that he has had several similar episodes in the past; however, this is the most severe the pain has ever been. On a scale of 1–10, with 10 being the most severe pain, the patient reports that the pain is a 9. He has been feeling nauseated since the onset of the pain and has had multiple episodes of vomiting. He denies diarrhea or constipation and states that vomiting seems to make his pain worse. He denies any fevers. When questioned about alcohol consumption the patient is evasive and answers that he occasionally drinks alcohol. Upon further questioning, the patient states that he drinks approximately three-fourth of a bottle of rum per day and has been doing so for the past 8 years. He smokes 1 pack of cigarettes per day. He lives with his wife and their two teenage daughters. He has no significant medical history.

Patient History Checklist

☐ Patient's name
☐ Patient's age
☐ Patient's address
☐ Patient's occupation
☐ Patient's presenting complaint
☐ Absence/presence of abdominal pain
☐ History of the pain
    ☐ Site
    ☐ Onset
    ☐ Duration

    ☐ Intensity
    ☐ Radiation
    ☐ Character
    ☐ Exacerbating factors
    ☐ Relieving factors
    ☐ Medications used to try to relieve the pain
☐ Previous episodes
☐ Presence of weight loss/gain
☐ Amount of weight loss/weight gain
☐ Time period of weight loss/weight gain
☐ Changes in bowel movements
☐ Changes in appetite (increased/decreased)
☐ Nausea/vomiting
☐ Presence of fever
☐ Presence of melena
☐ Presence of hematemesis
☐ Alcohol use (quantity/duration of use) (CAGE questions)
☐ Cigarette use (quantity/duration of use)
☐ Medical history
☐ Hospital admissions
☐ Surgical history
☐ Medications
☐ Family history
    ☐ Gastric ulcers
    ☐ Heart disease
    ☐ Diabetes
    ☐ Thyroid disease
    ☐ Cancer
    ☐ Others

Differential Diagnosis

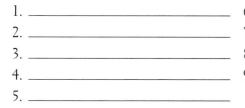
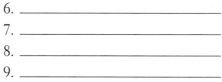

1. _____   6. _____
2. _____   7. _____
3. _____   8. _____
4. _____   9. _____
5. _____

Physical Examination Checklist

- ☐ Overall assessment
- ☐ Vitals
  - ☐ Temperature—assess for fever
  - ☐ Pulse—assess for tachycardia
  - ☐ Blood pressure—assess for hypotension or hypertension
  - ☐ Respirations
- ☐ Examine the abdomen
  - ☐ Inspect
  - ☐ Auscultate
  - ☐ Light palpation
  - ☐ Deep palpation
  - ☐ Assess for organomegaly (palpation and percussion)
  - ☐ Assess for muscular rigidity
  - ☐ Assess for rebound tenderness
  - ☐ Assess for fluid wave
  - ☐ Assess for shifting dullness
- ☐ Indicate to the patient that you would like to perform a digital rectal examination, but will not do so during this examination

Physical Examination Findings

General: 55-year-old male, very uncomfortable appearing. Noted to be sweating profusely throughout interview

Vitals:

Pulse—104/minute	Temperature—97.1°F
BP—158/96 mm Hg	Respirations—16/minute

Abdomen:

No ecchymosis visible

No visible masses

No striae noted

No visible peristalsis

Bowel sounds present in all quadrants

No bruits heard

No friction rubs over the spleen or liver

Marked tenderness to palpation in epigastric area

No hepatosplenomegaly

No rebound tenderness

No fluid wave noted

No shifting dullness noted

Differential Diagnosis

1. _____   3. _____
2. _____   4. _____

Follow-Up

1. _____   4. _____
2. _____   5. _____
3. _____

See Section III for differential diagnosis, appropriate follow-up, and brief case review.

CASE 9

A 34-year-old female is seen in the outpatient clinic with severe left-sided chest pain.

The patient also complains that she is having difficulty breathing. She finds that she is unable to catch her breath. The pain and the shortness of breath came on very suddenly approximately 2 hours prior to her visit to the clinic. The pain is constant and any movement seems to make the pain much worse. She also complains that she has had a cough for the past month following a flu and that every time she coughs or sneezes the pain is much worse. She has not been febrile at home. She denies nausea or vomiting. She feels like her heart is beating much faster than usual. She has never experienced these symptoms in the past. She has had no ill contacts and denies any recent travel out of the country. She lives at home with her husband and their two children, all of whom are well. Her medical history is unremarkable. She smokes about 10 cigarettes a day and denies the use of alcohol. She is currently taking an oral contraceptive medication.

Patient History Checklist

- ☐ Patient's name
- ☐ Patient's age
- ☐ Patient's address
- ☐ Patient's occupation
- ☐ Patient's presenting complaint
- ☐ Duration of symptoms
- ☐ Presence of cough (productive/nonproductive)
- ☐ Appearance of the sputum
- ☐ Presence of blood in the sputum
- ☐ Shortness of breath
- ☐ Presence of chest pain
- ☐ Time of onset of shortness of breath/chest pain

- ☐ Presence of fever
- ☐ Presence of diaphoresis
- ☐ Presence of rhinorrhea
- ☐ History of the pain
    - ☐ Site
    - ☐ Onset
    - ☐ Duration
    - ☐ Intensity
    - ☐ Radiation
    - ☐ Character
    - ☐ Exacerbating factors
    - ☐ Relieving factors
- ☐ Nausea/vomiting
- ☐ Recent illnesses
- ☐ History of weight loss
- ☐ Amount of weight loss
- ☐ Time period of weight loss
- ☐ Presence of night sweats
- ☐ Pain or swelling of the lower extremities
- ☐ Ill contacts
- ☐ Medical history
- ☐ Hospital admissions
- ☐ Surgical history
- ☐ Medications
- ☐ Family history
    - ☐ Cancer
    - ☐ Heart disease
    - ☐ Diabetes
    - ☐ Thyroid disease
    - ☐ Asthma/allergies
    - ☐ Others
- ☐ Social history
    - ☐ Smoking
    - ☐ Alcohol
    - ☐ Other drug use

Differential Diagnosis

1. _____   6. _____

2. _____   7. _____

3. _____   8. _____

4. _____   9. _____

5. _____

Physical Examination Checklist

☐ Overall assessment
☐ Vitals
    ☐ Temperature—assess for fever
    ☐ Pulse—assess for tachycardia
    ☐ Blood pressure
    ☐ Respirations—assess for tachypnea
☐ Examine the face
    ☐ Assess mucus membranes for the presence of cyanosis
☐ Examine the neck
    ☐ Assess for lymphadenopathy
    ☐ Assess for use of accessory muscles
    ☐ Assess the position of the trachea
☐ Examine the extremities
    ☐ Assess for clubbing
    ☐ Assess for cyanosis
☐ Respiratory system—examine the thorax
    ☐ Inspect
        ☐ Size
        ☐ Shape
        ☐ Symmetry
        ☐ Movement
        ☐ Deformities of the ribs
        ☐ Deformities of the spine
        ☐ Scars
    ☐ Palpate
        ☐ Tenderness

□ Excursion
□ Tactile fremitus
□ Chest dimensions
□ Position of the diaphragm
□ Percuss
□ All areas comparing side to side
□ Diaphragm excursion (left)
□ Diaphragm excursion (right)
□ Auscultate
□ All areas comparing side to side
□ Breath sounds
□ Vocal resonance
□ Whispering pectoriloquy
□ Aegophony
□ Perform a full cardiovascular examination, if time permits

Physical Examination Findings

General: 34-year-old female, uncomfortable appearing
Vitals:

    Pulse—102/minute   Temperature—98.1°F
    BP—122/84 mm Hg   Respirations—26/minute

HEENT:

    Mouth—Mucous membranes moist; no cyanosis noted

Neck:

    No lymphadenopathy
    Some use of accessory muscles of respirations
    Trachea midline

Extremities: No clubbing or cyanosis noted
Respiratory system:

    Thorax normal size and shape
    No asymmetry noted
    No scars or deformities noted

No tenderness to palpation
Tactile fremitus equal bilaterally
No increased anteroposterior diameter
Resonant to percussion bilaterally
Level of the diaphragms equal bilaterally
Breath sounds appreciated throughout
No wheezing noted
No whispering pectoriloquy noted
No aegophony noted

Differential Diagnosis

1. _____   3. _____
2. _____   4. _____

Follow-Up

1. _____   4. _____
2. _____   5. _____
3. _____

See Section III for differential diagnosis, appropriate follow-up, and brief case review.

CASE 10

A 45-year-old male is seen in the emergency department complaining of severe abdominal pain.

The pain is located in the upper abdomen, midline to slightly right-sided. The patient first had the pain upon waking up in the morning. He describes the pain as agonizing and "coming and going." He experiences the pain every 10 minutes. He denies fever. He has not had any constipation or diarrhea. His appetite was good until the onset of the pain this morning and since that time he has had nothing to eat. He has had a few similar episodes over the past year but the pain has never been as severe. He avoids fatty foods as they tend to make his stomach upset and the previous episodes have occurred following a greasy meal. He has no significant medical history. He has noticed that there has been a change in the color of his urine since waking up this morning—the urine is darker in color and appears frothy and bubbly. His family history is significant for gallbladder disease. Both his sister and his mother have had gallbladder surgery in the past. The only other significant family history is diabetes. The patient drinks approximately four beers a night and smokes approximately 15 cigarettes a day.

Patient History Checklist

- ☐ Patient's name
- ☐ Patient's age
- ☐ Patient's address
- ☐ Patient's occupation
- ☐ Patient's presenting complaint.
- ☐ Absence/presence of abdominal pain
- ☐ History of the pain
  - ☐ Site
  - ☐ Onset
  - ☐ Duration

- ☐ Intensity
- ☐ Radiation
- ☐ Character
- ☐ Exacerbating factors
- ☐ Relieving factors
☐ Changes in bowel movements
☐ Change in color of stool
☐ Changes in appetite (increased/decreased)
☐ Changes in diet
☐ Presence of weight loss/gain
☐ Amount of weight loss/weight gain
☐ Time period of weight loss/weight gain
☐ Presence of nausea/vomiting
☐ Change in color of urine
☐ Previous episodes
☐ Medical history
☐ Hospital admissions
☐ Surgical history
☐ Medications
☐ Family history
- ☐ Gallbladder disease
- ☐ Heart disease
- ☐ Diabetes
- ☐ Thyroid disease
- ☐ Cancer
- ☐ Others
☐ Social history
- ☐ Smoking
- ☐ Alcohol
- ☐ Other drug use

Differential Diagnosis

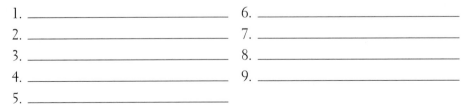

1. _____   6. _____
2. _____   7. _____
3. _____   8. _____
4. _____   9. _____
5. _____

Physical Examination Checklist

☐ Overall assessment
☐ Vitals
    ☐ Temperature—assess for fever
    ☐ Pulse—assess for tachycardia
    ☐ Blood pressure—assess for hypotension
    ☐ Respirations
☐ Examine the abdomen
    ☐ Inspect
    ☐ Auscultate
    ☐ Light palpation
    ☐ Deep palpation
    ☐ Assess for organomegaly (palpation and percussion)
    ☐ Assess for muscular rigidity
    ☐ Assess for rebound tenderness
    ☐ Murphy's sign
    ☐ Boas' sign
    ☐ Assess for fluid wave
    ☐ Assess for shifting dullness
☐ Indicate to the patient that you would like to perform a rectal examination, but will not do so during this examination

Physical Examination Findings

General: 45-year-old male, uncomfortable appearing
Vitals:

Pulse—96/minute   Temperature—97.9°F
BP—136/92 mm Hg   Respirations—18/minute

Abdomen:

No ecchymosis visible
No visible masses
No striae noted
No visible peristalsis
Bowel sounds present in all quadrants

No bruits heard

No friction rubs over the spleen or liver

Marked tenderness to palpation in right upper quadrant

No hepatosplenomegaly

No rebound tenderness

Murphy's sign positive

Boas' sign positive

No fluid wave appreciated

No shifting dullness appreciated

Differential Diagnosis

1. _____   3. _____
2. _____   4. _____

Follow-Up

1. _____   4. _____
2. _____   5. _____
3. _____

See Section III for differential diagnosis, appropriate follow-up, and brief case review.

CASE 11

A 68-year-old female is brought to the family physician by her husband. He has noticed that she is having increasing difficulty with her memory.

The patient's husband states that it seems to be mainly her short-term memory that is affected. She is able to recall events that happened many years ago in detail, but is often unable to recall something that happened earlier the same day or earlier in the week. She denies this and states that her memory is just fine. Her husband has also been noticing that she often calls objects by the wrong names. She has been healthy in the past. Her medical history is significant for hypothyroidism, which she was diagnosed with 10 years ago. The only medication she uses is thyroxine for the hypothyroidism. She has no allergies. She denies the use of alcohol or any other drug use.

Patient History Checklist

☐ Patient's name
☐ Patient's age
☐ Patient's address
☐ Patient's occupation
☐ Patient's presenting complaint
☐ Duration of symptoms
☐ Presence of memory loss
☐ Presence of forgetfulness
☐ Difficulty concentrating
☐ Presence of fatigue
☐ Presence of irritability
☐ Difficulty sleeping
☐ Loss of appetite
☐ Presence of weight loss/gain
☐ Amount of weight loss/weight gain
☐ Time period of weight loss/weight gain

- ☐ Presence of hallucinations
- ☐ Altered level of consciousness
- ☐ Presence of delusions
- ☐ Previous episode of symptoms
- ☐ Heat intolerance
- ☐ Palpitations
- ☐ Anxiety
- ☐ Cold intolerance
- ☐ Medical history
- ☐ Hospital admissions
- ☐ Surgical history
- ☐ Medications
- ☐ Family history
  - ☐ Psychiatric illnesses
  - ☐ Heart disease
  - ☐ Diabetes
  - ☐ Thyroid disease
  - ☐ Cancer
  - ☐ Others
- ☐ Social history
  - ☐ Smoking
  - ☐ Alcohol
  - ☐ Other drug use
  - ☐ Family situation
  - ☐ Work situation
  - ☐ Ability to function at work
  - ☐ Ability to function at home
  - ☐ Presence of support system
  - ☐ Ability to perform daily tasks
  - ☐ Ability to safely reside at home

Differential Diagnosis

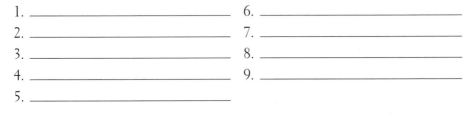

1. _____ 6. _____
2. _____ 7. _____
3. _____ 8. _____
4. _____ 9. _____
5. _____

Physical Examination Checklist

☐ Overall assessment
☐ Vitals
   ☐ Temperature
   ☐ Pulse
      ☐ Assess for tachycardia or bradycardia
      ☐ Assess for arrhythmias
   ☐ Blood pressure
   ☐ Respirations
☐ Evaluate mental status
   ☐ Orientation to person, place, and time
   ☐ Level of consciousness
   ☐ Short-term memory
   ☐ Long-term memory
   ☐ Observe the patient's gait and speech
☐ Examine the head
   ☐ Assess for masses, ecchymosis, lacerations, tenderness
☐ Examine the ears
   ☐ Assess the external ear canal for fluid drainage
   ☐ Assess the tympanic membranes
☐ Examine all cranial nerves (I–XII)
☐ Examine the sensory system
   ☐ Check for pain and crude touch in all parts of the body
   ☐ Romberg's test
   ☐ Proprioception at fingers and toes
   ☐ Vibratory sense
   ☐ Stereognosis
   ☐ Graphesthesia
   ☐ 2-point discrimination
   ☐ Point localization
   ☐ Extinction
☐ Examine the motor system
   ☐ Inspect the motor system for atrophy, fasciculations, and involuntary movements
   ☐ Palpate all limbs for muscle tone
   ☐ Check all major muscle groups for power
   ☐ Check all reflexes

☐ Abdominal
☐ Plantar
☐ Biceps
☐ Triceps
☐ Brachioradialis
☐ Knee
☐ Ankle
☐ Examine the cerebellum
   ☐ Ask the patient to walk in a straight line, heel to toe
   ☐ Ask the patient to walk in a straight line on his/her heels
   ☐ Ask the patient to walk in a straight line on his/her toes
   ☐ Ask the patient to perform the finger–nose test
   ☐ Ask the patient to perform the knee–heel–shin test
   ☐ Check for dysdiadochokinesia

Physical Examination Findings

General: 68-year-old female, no acute distress
Vitals:

Pulse—78/minute	Temperature—98.8°F
BP—134/84 mm Hg	Respirations—16/minute

Mental status:

Patient oriented to person
Not oriented to place or time
Patient awake and alert
Long-term memory intact
Short-term memory impaired
No abnormal gait observed
Speech appropriate

HEENT:

Head—No masses, ecchymosis, lacerations, or tenderness appreciated
Ears—No drainage noted; tympanic membranes visualized bilaterally

Cranial nerves: I–XII intact

Sensory system: Sensation intact bilaterally

Motor system:

    No atrophy noted

    No fasciculations

    Normal muscle tone noted in all extremities

    Normal power observed in all extremities

    Deep tendon reflexes intact

    Abdominal reflex present

    Plantar reflex down going

Cerebellum: No abnormalities noted

Differential Diagnosis

1. _____   3. _____
2. _____   4. _____

Follow-Up

1. _____   4. _____
2. _____   5. _____
3. _____

See Section III for differential diagnosis, appropriate follow-up, and brief case review.

A 21-year-old female phones you concerning her newborn infant who has a fever.

The infant is now 5 weeks old. The patient's mother states that she is worried about germs in the clinic and so decided not to bring the infant to the clinic for fear that he would come into contact with infection. The infant she reports is not doing too well. He has been healthy since birth until yesterday when he developed a fever. She reports that he has been feeding well and gaining weight until the onset of the fever. He is both breast and bottle fed. His bowel movements have been regular. The maximum temperature (rectally) at home was 102.5°F. He has had one episode of vomiting and has not been eating well since the onset. She has noticed that he has had fewer wet diapers than usual over the past 24 hours. The infant lives at home with his mother, his father, and 1 sibling (3 years old), and they are all well. She has not noticed any skin rashes. His delivery was a normal vaginal delivery and there were no complications during the pregnancy.

Patient History Checklist

- ☐ Patient's name
- ☐ Patient's age
- ☐ Patient's address
- ☐ Patient's presenting complaint
- ☐ Maximum temperature
- ☐ Presence of weight loss/gain
- ☐ Amount of weight loss/weight gain
- ☐ Time period of weight loss/weight gain
- ☐ Changes in bowel movements
- ☐ Changes in appetite (increased/decreased)
- ☐ Number of wet diapers
- ☐ Presence of skin rash
- ☐ Irritability/lethargy

☐ Presence of cough
☐ Presence of shortness of breath
☐ Ill contacts (especially household members)
☐ Birth history
　☐ Weeks of gestation at delivery
　☐ Complications during the pregnancy
　☐ Frequency of prenatal care
　☐ Duration of labor
　☐ Complications during delivery
　☐ Mother tested for group B strep
　☐ Mother treated for group B strep (if necessary)
　☐ Immunizations up to date
　☐ Mother's prior pregnancies
　☐ Outcomes of any prior pregnancies
☐ Family history of diseases (mother, father, and siblings)
　☐ Heart disease
　☐ Diabetes
　☐ Thyroid disease
　☐ Sickle-cell disease
　☐ Psychiatric disorders
　☐ Sexually transmitted diseases
☐ Diet (breast or bottle fed)
☐ Social history
　☐ Living situation
　☐ Pets in the home
　☐ Smoking in the home

Differential Diagnosis

1. _____   6. _____
2. _____   7. _____
3. _____   8. _____
4. _____   9. _____
5. _____

Physical Examination Checklist

Advise the mother to bring the infant to the clinic for a full assessment. If the history suggests that the infant requires hospitalization, advise the mother to take the infant to the emergency department immediately for evaluation.

Follow-Up

1. _____   4. _____

2. _____   5. _____

3. _____

See Section III for differential diagnosis, appropriate follow-up, and brief case review.

A 22-year-old female is brought to the emergency department by her stepfather, who complains of her recent strange behavior . He feels that his stepdaughter is confused and delusional.

Upon asking the patient some questions, it is discovered that she has been having some paranoid delusions regarding some of the members of the church in which she is involved. She states that the other members of the church whisper behind her back and are plotting against her. She also states that she is quite sure that her mother and her stepfather are also in on the plan and that she cannot trust them to help her. She states that there is nothing wrong with her and feels that her stepfather bringing her to the emergency department is all part of the same sinister plan against her. She goes on to say that these people can't hurt her because she is well protected by Jesus. She states that Jesus has placed a shield around her, protecting her from them. Past history suggests that the patient did not do well in school, had very few friends, and spent most of the time by herself. She smokes approximately one and half packs of cigarettes per day and admits that she occasionally drinks alcohol, but will not quantify how much or how often she drinks.

Patient History Checklist

☐ Patient's name
☐ Patient's age
☐ Patient's address
☐ Patient's occupation
☐ Patient's presenting complaint
☐ Duration of symptoms
☐ Presence of irritability
☐ Difficulty concentrating
☐ Presence of hallucinations
☐ Presence of delusions

- ☐ Presence of disorganized thinking
- ☐ Presence of agitation
- ☐ Lack of initiative
- ☐ Lack of emotional responses
- ☐ Difficulty sleeping
- ☐ Loss of appetite
- ☐ Presence of weight loss/gain
- ☐ Amount of weight loss/weight gain
- ☐ Time period of weight loss/weight gain
- ☐ Previous episode of symptoms
- ☐ Suicidal ideation
    - ☐ Suicide plan
    - ☐ Previous suicide attempts
- ☐ Homicidal ideation
- ☐ Medical history
- ☐ Hospital admissions
- ☐ Surgical history
- ☐ Medications
- ☐ Family history
    - ☐ Psychiatric illnesses
    - ☐ Depression
    - ☐ Heart disease
    - ☐ Diabetes
    - ☐ Thyroid disease
    - ☐ Cancer
    - ☐ Others
- ☐ Social history
    - ☐ Smoking
    - ☐ Alcohol (CAGE questions)
    - ☐ Other drug use
    - ☐ Family situation
    - ☐ Work situation
    - ☐ Ability to function at work
    - ☐ Ability to function at home
    - ☐ Presence of support system

Differential Diagnosis

1. _____   6. _____
2. _____   7. _____
3. _____   8. _____
4. _____   9. _____
5. _____

Physical Examination Checklist

☐ Evaluate mental status
  ☐ Orientation to person, place, and time
  ☐ Level of consciousness
  ☐ Short-term memory
  ☐ Long-term memory
  ☐ Abstract or concrete thinking
  ☐ Mood and affect
☐ Observe the patient's gait and speech
☐ Perform a complete physical examination, if time permits

Physical Examination Findings

General: 22-year-old female, no acute distress. Patient agitated and nervous appearing during interview. Her clothes are disheveled and her hair is unkempt.

Vitals:

Pulse—94/minute   Temperature—98.2°F

BP—138/88 mm Hg   Respirations—16/minute

Mental status:

Patient oriented to person, place, and time

Patient awake and alert

Long-term memory unable to assess—patient uncooperative

Short-term memory impaired

No abnormal gait observed
Speech appropriate
Patient experiencing hallucinations and delusions
Patient experiencing paranoia

Differential Diagnosis

1. _____   3. _____
2. _____   4. _____

Follow-Up

1. _____   4. _____
2. _____   5. _____
3. _____

See Section III for differential diagnosis, appropriate follow-up, and brief case review.

CASE 14

A 26-year-old female is seen by her primary care physician complaining of a headache.

The headache started early in the morning. She describes the pain as throbbing and localized to her right side. She also reports that she is having difficulty dealing with bright lights and finds that if she lies still in a dark room the pain subsides slightly. She has vomited twice since the onset of the pain. She has had many of these headaches in the past. The first time that she ever experienced a headache similar to this one was at the age of 14. She has about 3–4 such headaches per year and finds that they are closely related to stress. She has just divorced her husband after only 1 year of marriage and is feeling very depressed and stressed about the whole divorce settlement. She has no other health problems and does not take any medications.

Patient History Checklist

- ☐ Patient's name
- ☐ Patient's age
- ☐ Patient's address
- ☐ Patient's occupation
- ☐ Patient's presenting complaint
- ☐ Absence/presence pain
- ☐ History of the pain
  - ☐ Site
  - ☐ Onset
  - ☐ Duration
  - ☐ Intensity
  - ☐ Radiation
  - ☐ Character
  - ☐ Exacerbating factors
  - ☐ Relieving factors
  - ☐ Medications used to relieve symptoms

☐ Changes in vision
☐ Presence of dizziness
☐ Presence of nausea/vomiting
☐ Presence of fatigue
☐ Presence of irritability
☐ Difficulty concentrating
☐ Difficulty sleeping
☐ Previous episode of symptoms
☐ History of trauma
☐ Medical history
☐ Hospital admissions
☐ Surgical history
☐ Medications
☐ Family history
    ☐ Heart disease
    ☐ Diabetes
    ☐ Thyroid disease
    ☐ Cancer
    ☐ Psychiatric illnesses
    ☐ Others

Differential Diagnosis

1. _____   6. _____
2. _____   7. _____
3. _____   8. _____
4. _____   9. _____
5. _____

Physical Examination Checklist

☐ Overall assessment
☐ Vitals
    ☐ Temperature—assess for fever
    ☐ Pulse

- [ ] Blood pressure
- [ ] Respirations
- [ ] Evaluate mental status
  - [ ] Orientation to person, place, and time
  - [ ] Level of consciousness
  - [ ] Short-term memory
  - [ ] Long-term memory
  - [ ] Observe the patient's gait and speech
- [ ] Examine the head
  - [ ] Assess for masses, ecchymosis, lacerations, tenderness
- [ ] Examine the eyes
  - [ ] Assess for papilledema
- [ ] Examine the ears
  - [ ] Assess the external ear canal for fluid drainage
  - [ ] Assess the tympanic membranes
- [ ] Assess for cervical rigidity
- [ ] Brudzinski's sign
- [ ] Kernig's sign
- [ ] Examine all cranial nerves (I–XII)
- [ ] Examine the sensory system
  - [ ] Check for pain and crude touch in all parts of the body
  - [ ] Romberg's test
  - [ ] Proprioception at fingers and toes
  - [ ] Vibratory sense
  - [ ] Stereognosis
  - [ ] Graphesthesia
  - [ ] 2-point discrimination
  - [ ] Point localization
  - [ ] Extinction
- [ ] Examine the motor system
  - [ ] Inspect the motor system for atrophy, fasciculations, and involuntary movements
  - [ ] Palpate all limbs for muscle tone
  - [ ] Check all major muscle groups for power
- [ ] Check all reflexes
  - [ ] Abdominal
  - [ ] Plantar
  - [ ] Biceps

   □ Triceps
   □ Brachioradialis
   □ Knee
   □ Ankle
□ Examine the cerebellum
   □ Ask the patient to walk in a straight line, heel to toes
   □ Ask the patient to walk in a straight line on his/her heels
   □ Ask the patient to walk in a straight line on his/her toes
   □ Ask the patient to perform the finger–nose test
   □ Ask the patient to perform the knee–heel–shin test
   □ Check for dysdiadochokinesia

Physical Examination Findings

General: 26-year-old female, no acute distress

Vitals:

   Pulse—68/minute   Temperature—97.6°F

   BP—112/72 mm Hg   Respirations—14/minute

Mental status:

   Patient oriented to person, place, and time

   Short and long-term memory intact

   No abnormal gait observed

   Speech appropriate

HEENT:

   Head—No masses, ecchymosis, lacerations, or tenderness appreciated

   Eyes—No papilledema noted on fundoscopy

   Ears—No drainage noted; tympanic membranes visualized bilaterally

   No cervical rigidity appreciated

   Brudzinski's sign negative

   Kernig's sign negative

Cranial nerves: I–XII intact

Sensory system: Sensation intact bilaterally

Motor system:
  No atrophy noted
  No fasciculations
  Normal muscle tone noted in all extremities
  Normal power observed in all extremities
  Deep tendon reflexes intact
  Abdominal reflex present
  Plantar reflex down going
Cerebellum: No abnormalities noted

Differential Diagnosis

1. _____   3. _____
2. _____   4. _____

Follow-Up

1. _____   4. _____
2. _____   5. _____
3. _____

See Section III for differential diagnosis, appropriate follow-up, and brief case review.

A 27-year-old female is seen in the clinic complaining of chest pain.

The patient complains that the pain is on the left side of her chest and is particularly painful when she takes a deep breath or presses on the area. She states that she had a fall at home but is vague about the details of how the fall came about. She lives at home with her husband and their three children. She is a stay-at-home mom. When questioned about her medical history she is again vague and states that she has been healthy with the exception of some bruises, broken bones, and lacerations from previous falls. She has been seen in the emergency department seven times in the past year for injuries. In the past she has sustained a broken jaw, a broken left fibula, and multiple rib fractures. When questioned about her married life, the patient becomes tearful and upset. She states that the only reason that she is attending the clinic is to obtain something for the pain in her side and that there are no further issues that she would like to discuss.

Patient History Checklist

- ☐ Patient's name
- ☐ Patient's age
- ☐ Patient's address
- ☐ Patient's occupation
- ☐ Patient's presenting complaint
- ☐ Presence of chest pain
- ☐ Site of chest pain
- ☐ History of the pain
  - ☐ Site
  - ☐ Onset etc.
- ☐ Presence of ecchymosis
- ☐ Duration of symptoms
- ☐ Previous episode of symptoms
- ☐ Shortness of breath

- [ ] Severity of the symptoms
- [ ] Relieving factors
- [ ] Aggravating factors
- [ ] Medications used during this acute episode/effect of medications used
- [ ] Abuse history
  - [ ] How injury occurred
  - [ ] Presence of abuse in the home
  - [ ] History of abuse in the home
  - [ ] Frequency of abuse
  - [ ] Presence of emotional abuse
  - [ ] Presence of physical abuse
  - [ ] Presence of sexual abuse
  - [ ] Presence of child abuse in the home
  - [ ] Presence of guns in the home
  - [ ] Use of alcohol in the home
  - [ ] Use of illegal drugs in the home
  - [ ] Presence of an escape plan
- [ ] Medical history
- [ ] Hospital admissions
- [ ] Surgical history
- [ ] Medications
- [ ] Family history
  - [ ] Depression
  - [ ] Psychiatric illnesses
  - [ ] Heart disease
  - [ ] Diabetes
  - [ ] Thyroid disease
  - [ ] Cancer
  - [ ] Others
- [ ] Social history
  - [ ] Smoking
  - [ ] Alcohol
  - [ ] Other drug use
  - [ ] Family situation
  - [ ] Work situation
  - [ ] Ability to function at work
  - [ ] Ability to function at home
  - [ ] Presence of support system

Differential Diagnosis

1. _____   6. _____
2. _____   7. _____
3. _____   8. _____
4. _____   9. _____
5. _____

Physical Examination Checklist

- ☐ Overall assessment
- ☐ Vitals
  - ☐ Temperature
  - ☐ Pulse
  - ☐ Blood pressure
  - ☐ Respirations
- ☐ Respiratory system — examine the thorax
  - ☐ Inspect
    - ☐ Size
    - ☐ Shape
    - ☐ Symmetry
    - ☐ Movement
    - ☐ Deformities of the ribs
    - ☐ Deformities of the spine
    - ☐ Scars
  - ☐ Palpate
    - ☐ Tenderness
    - ☐ Excursion
    - ☐ Tactile fremitus
    - ☐ Chest dimensions
    - ☐ Position of the diaphragm
  - ☐ Percuss
    - ☐ All areas comparing side to side
    - ☐ Diaphragm excursion (left)
    - ☐ Diaphragm excursion (right)

    ☐ Auscultate
        ☐ All areas comparing side to side
        ☐ Breath sounds
        ☐ Vocal resonance
        ☐ Whispering pectoriloquy
        ☐ Aegophony
    ☐ Examine the skin
        ☐ Assess for areas of ecchymosis, lacerations, and scars
    ☐ Perform a complete physical examination, if time permits, to assess for other signs of physical abuse

Physical Examination Findings

General: 27-year-old female, mildly agitated
Vitals:

Pulse—94/minute	Temperature—97.7°F
BP—134/90 mm Hg	Respirations—18/minute

Respiratory system:

Thorax normal size and shape

No asymmetry noted

No scars or deformities noted

Small ecchymosis noted on lower left side of chest

Tenderness to palpation on lower left side of chest

Excursion equal bilaterally

Tactile fremitus equal bilaterally

No increased anteroposterior diameter

Resonant to percussion bilaterally

Level of the diaphragms equal bilaterally

Breath sounds appreciated throughout

No wheezing noted

No whispering pectoriloquy noted

No aegophony noted

Skin: Small ecchymosis noted on left anterior thigh and larger ecchymosis noted on right posterior thigh

Differential Diagnosis

1. _____   3. _____
2. _____   4. _____

Follow-Up

1. _____   4. _____
2. _____   5. _____
3. _____

See Section III for differential diagnosis, appropriate follow-up, and brief case review.

CASE 16

A 16-year-old male is brought to the outpatient department by his mother. He has been experiencing shortness of breath for the past 3 days.

His mother states that he has been asthmatic since the age of 2. The patient usually suffers two to three asthma attacks per year. He is allergic to cat dander and also to dust. Three days ago he began to feel short of breath and was noticed by his mother to be wheezing. He has been using his inhaler since that time with some relief. He states that he is still short of breath on exertion and is still waking up a few times in the night feeling uncomfortable and having to use his inhaler. He has no other significant medical history and his family history is unremarkable.

Patient History Checklist

☐ Patient's name
☐ Patient's age
☐ Patient's address
☐ Patient's occupation
☐ Patient's presenting complaint
☐ Duration of symptoms
☐ Presence of cough (productive/nonproductive)
☐ Appearance of the sputum
☐ Presence of fever
☐ Shortness of breath
☐ Severity of the symptoms
☐ Relieving factors
☐ Aggravating factors
☐ Medications used during this acute episode/effect of medications used
☐ Presence of chest pain
☐ Presence of rhinorrhea
☐ Allergies

☐ Frequency of attacks
☐ Prior hospitalizations for asthma
☐ Asthma triggers
☐ Medical history
☐ Hospital admissions
☐ Surgical history
☐ Medications
☐ Family history
    ☐ Asthma/allergies
    ☐ Heart disease
    ☐ Diabetes
    ☐ Thyroid disease
    ☐ Cancer
    ☐ Others
☐ Social history
    ☐ Smoking
    ☐ Alcohol
    ☐ Other drug use
    ☐ Occupational exposure to dust inhalation

Differential Diagnosis

1. _____   6. _____
2. _____   7. _____
3. _____   8. _____
4. _____   9. _____
5. _____

Physical Examination Checklist

☐ Overall assessment
☐ Vitals
    ☐ Temperature
    ☐ Pulse—assess for tachycardia
    ☐ Blood pressure
    ☐ Respirations—assess for tachypnea

- ☐ Examine the face
  - ☐ Assess mucus membranes for the presence of cyanosis or pallor
- ☐ Examine the extremities
  - ☐ Assess for clubbing
  - ☐ Assess for cyanosis
- ☐ Examine the neck
  - ☐ Assess for lymphadenopathy
  - ☐ Assess for use of accessory muscles of respiration
  - ☐ Assess the position of the trachea
- ☐ Respiratory system—examine the thorax
  - ☐ Inspect
    - ☐ Size
    - ☐ Shape
    - ☐ Symmetry
    - ☐ Movement
    - ☐ Deformities of the ribs
    - ☐ Deformities of the spine
    - ☐ Scars
  - ☐ Palpate
    - ☐ Tenderness
    - ☐ Excursion
    - ☐ Tactile fremitus
    - ☐ Chest dimensions
    - ☐ Position of the diaphragm
  - ☐ Percuss
    - ☐ All areas comparing side to side
    - ☐ Diaphragm excursion (left)
    - ☐ Diaphragm excursion (right)
  - ☐ Auscultate
    - ☐ All areas comparing side to side
    - ☐ Breath sounds
    - ☐ Vocal resonance
    - ☐ Whispering pectoriloquy
    - ☐ Aegophony

Physical Examination Findings

General: 16-year-old male in mild distress
Vitals:

    Pulse—94/minute   Temperature—97.7°F

    BP—120/80 mm Hg   Respirations—24/minute

HEENT:

    Mouth—Mucous membranes moist; No cyanosis noted

Extremities: No clubbing or cyanosis noted
Neck:

    No lymphadenopathy

    Some use of accessory muscles of respirations

    Trachea midline

Respiratory system:

    Thorax normal size and shape

    No asymmetry noted

    No scars or deformities noted

    No tenderness to palpation

    Excursion equal bilaterally

    Tactile fremitus equal bilaterally

    No increased anteroposterior diameter

    Resonant to percussion bilaterally

    Level of the diaphragms equal bilaterally

    Breath sounds appreciated throughout

    Mild expiratory wheezing noted throughout lung fields

    No vocal resonance noted

    No whispering pectoriloquy noted

    No aegophony noted

Differential Diagnosis

1. _____   3. _____
2. _____   4. _____

Follow-Up

1. _____   4. _____
2. _____   5. _____
3. _____

See Section III for differential diagnosis, appropriate follow-up, and brief case review.

CASE 17

A 54-year-old female complains of fatigue and dizziness for the past 2 weeks.

The patient has also been feeling very sweaty and a little faint upon standing up. She has been having loose stools for the past 2 weeks, approximately three to five stools per day. She has noticed that the color of her stool seems to have changed and her stool is now very dark in color, almost black. She denies ever seeing any bright red blood in her stool. She has been healthy in the past with the exception of frequent indigestion which is usually relieved by antacids or a large glass of milk. She lives with her husband and her two daughters, all of whom are healthy. She smokes approximately 1 pack of cigarettes per day and admits to drinking between three to five vodkas per day. Her family history is unremarkable.

Patient History Checklist

- ☐ Patient's name
- ☐ Patient's age
- ☐ Patient's address
- ☐ Patient's occupation
- ☐ Patient's presenting complaint
- ☐ Absence/presence of abdominal pain
- ☐ Pain in relation to meals
- ☐ Changes in bowel movements
- ☐ Changes in appetite (increased/decreased)
- ☐ Presence of weight loss/gain
- ☐ Amount of weight loss/weight gain
- ☐ Time period of weight loss/weight gain
- ☐ Presence of dizziness
- ☐ Presence of lightheadedness
- ☐ Presence of fatigue
- ☐ Presence of melena

☐ Presence of hematemesis
☐ History of gastric ulcers
☐ History of hemorrhoids
☐ Last menstrual period
☐ Medications taken to relieve symptoms
☐ Medical history
☐ Hospital admissions
☐ Surgical history
☐ Medications
☐ Family history
   ☐ Colon cancer
   ☐ Diabetes
   ☐ Thyroid disease
   ☐ Others
☐ Social history
   ☐ Smoking
   ☐ Alcohol (CAGE questions)
   ☐ Other drug use

Differential Diagnosis

1. _____   6. _____
2. _____   7. _____
3. _____   8. _____
4. _____   9. _____
5. _____

Physical Examination Checklist

☐ Overall assessment
☐ Vitals
   ☐ Temperature
   ☐ Pulse—assess for tachycardia
   ☐ Blood pressure—assess for postural hypotension
   ☐ Respirations

☐ Examine the abdomen
   ☐ Inspect
   ☐ Auscultate
   ☐ Light palpation
   ☐ Deep palpation
   ☐ Assess for organomegaly (palpation and percussion)
   ☐ Assess for muscular rigidity
   ☐ Assess for rebound tenderness
☐ Indicate to the patient that you would like to perform a digital rectal exami-
   nation but will not do so during this examination

Physical Examination Findings

General: 54-year-old female, uncomfortable appearing
Vitals:

   Pulse—97/minute   Temperature—98.8°F
   BP—104/64 mm Hg   Respirations—12/minute

Abdomen:

   No ecchymosis visible
   No visible masses
   No striae noted
   No visible peristalsis
   Bowel sounds present in all quadrants
   No bruits heard
   No friction rubs over the spleen or liver
   No tenderness to palpation
   No hepatosplenomegaly
   No rebound tenderness

Differential Diagnosis

1. _____   3. _____
2. _____   4. _____

Follow-Up

1. _____   4. _____

2. _____   5. _____

3. _____

See Section III for differential diagnosis, appropriate follow-up, and brief case review.

CASE 18

A 56-year-old male is seen by his primary care physician for follow-up care of his diabetes.

The patient is a known diabetic and follows up with his physician every 3 months for care of his diabetes. He was first diagnosed with diabetes 6 years ago. He has had no diabetic complications to date and his blood sugar is well controlled. He checks his blood glucose at home three times per day. He has no other medical conditions and has been well in the past. He is obese, but he has been maintaining a steady weight for the past 3 years. His family history is significant for heart disease, hypertension, and diabetes. He denies the use of alcohol and cigarettes.

Patient History Checklist

☐ Patient's name
☐ Patient's age
☐ Patient's address
☐ Patient's occupation
☐ Patient's presenting complaint
☐ Presence of polyuria
☐ Presence of polydipsia
☐ Presence of excessive thirst
☐ Blood glucose readings at home
☐ Diet
☐ Presence of weight loss/gain
☐ Amount of weight loss/weight gain
☐ Time period of weight loss/weight gain
☐ Presence of chest pain
☐ Presence of shortness of breath
☐ Presence of peripheral edema
☐ Changes in vision

☐ Presence of lower extremity ulcers or sores
☐ Family history
   ☐ Heart disease
   ☐ Diabetes
   ☐ Hypertension
   ☐ Previous heart condition
   ☐ Smoking
   ☐ Alcohol
   ☐ Exercise
   ☐ Occupation
   ☐ Stress at present
☐ Medical history
☐ Hospital admissions
☐ Surgical history
☐ Medications

Differential Diagnosis

1. _____   6. _____
2. _____   7. _____
3. _____   8. _____
4. _____   9. _____
5. _____

Physical Examination Checklist

☐ Overall assessment
☐ Vitals
   ☐ Temperature
   ☐ Pulse
   ☐ Blood pressure
   ☐ Respirations
☐ Examine the eyes (especially fundoscopy)
   ☐ Cataract
   ☐ Retinal hemorrhages
   ☐ Microaneurysms

- ☐ Neovascularization
- ☐ Hard exudates
- ☐ Examine the neck
  - ☐ Examine JVP wave pattern
  - ☐ Measure the JVP
  - ☐ Assess hepatojugular reflux
  - ☐ Carotid arteries—assess for bruits
- ☐ Cardiovascular system
  - ☐ Inspect the precordium
  - ☐ Shape
  - ☐ Scars
  - ☐ Pulses
  - ☐ Apex
- ☐ Palpate the precordium
  - ☐ Tenderness
  - ☐ Pulses
  - ☐ Apex
  - ☐ Thrills
  - ☐ Heaves
- ☐ Percuss the heart borders
- ☐ Auscultate with the bell
  - ☐ Aortic area
  - ☐ Pulmonic area
  - ☐ Erb's point
  - ☐ Tricuspid area
  - ☐ Apex (mitral) area
- ☐ Auscultate with the diaphragm
  - ☐ Aortic area
  - ☐ Pulmonic area
  - ☐ Erb's point
  - ☐ Tricuspid area
  - ☐ Apex (mitral) area
- ☐ Auscultate with the bell—patient in left lateral recumbent position
- ☐ Auscultate with the diaphragm—patient in aortic position
- ☐ Inspect the upper and lower extremities for size and symmetry
- ☐ Examine the nails, hair, and skin
- ☐ Observe any ulcers or gangrene, taking care to examine the soles of the feet

☐ Palpate temperature in both the upper and the lower extremities comparing both limbs
☐ Palpate pulses
   ☐ Dorsalis pedis
   ☐ Posterior tibial
   ☐ Popliteal
   ☐ Femoral
   ☐ Radial
   ☐ Ulnar
   ☐ Brachial
☐ Perform Allen's test
☐ Perform Buerger's test
☐ Check for bruits over the abdominal aorta and both the iliofemoral arteries
☐ Examine the motor system
   ☐ Inspect the motor system for atrophy, fasciculations, and involuntary movements
   ☐ Palpate all limbs for muscle tone
   ☐ Check all major muscle groups for power
   ☐ Check all reflexes
      ☐ Abdominal
      ☐ Plantar
      ☐ Biceps
      ☐ Triceps
      ☐ Brachioradialis
      ☐ Knee
      ☐ Ankle
☐ Examine the sensory system
   ☐ Check for pain and crude touch in all parts of the body
   ☐ Romberg's test
   ☐ Proprioception at fingers and toes
   ☐ Vibratory sense
   ☐ Stereognosis
   ☐ Graphesthesia
   ☐ 2-point discrimination
   ☐ Point localization
   ☐ Extinction

Physical Examination Findings

General: 56-year-old male, no acute distress
Vitals:

Pulse—76/minute	Temperature—97.4°F
BP—124/80 mm Hg	Respirations—12/minute

Eyes:

No asymmetry noted

No lid swellings, lesions, or retractions noted

Visual acuity 20/20 in left eye, 20/20 in right eye, 20/20 in both eyes

No peripheral field deficits noted

No lens opacities noted

Pupils equal and reactive to light and accommodation bilaterally

No retinal hemorrhages, microaneurysms, neovascularization, or hard exudates noted

Neck:

No JVP noted

No hepatojugular reflux noted

No carotid bruits appreciated

Cardiovascular system:

Precordium normal shape and size

No abnormal pulsations appreciated

Apical, suprasternal, and abdominal pulsations observed

No tenderness to palpation

Apical, suprasternal, and abdominal pulsations all palpable

No thrills or heaves

S1, S2 heard, no murmurs

Upper extremities:

Symmetrical

Temperature equal bilaterally

No ecchymosis, erythema, swellings, or deformities noted

No tenderness on palpation

No ulcers or gangrene noted

Normal hair distribution

No thickening or ridges of the nails

Lower Extremities:

Symmetrical

Temperature equal bilaterally

No ecchymosis, erythema, swellings, or deformities noted

No tenderness on palpation

No ulcers or gangrene noted

Normal hair distribution

No thickening or ridges of the nails

All peripheral pulses palpable

Allen's test negative

Buerger's test negative

No bruits noted over abdominal aorta or iliofemoral arteries

Motor system:

No atrophy noted

No fasciculations

Normal muscle tone noted in all extremities

Normal power observed in all extremities

Deep tendon reflexes intact

Abdominal reflex present

Plantar reflex down going

Sensory system: Sensation intact bilaterally

Differential Diagnosis

1. _____   3. _____
2. _____   4. _____

Follow-Up

1. _____   4. _____

2. _____   5. _____

3. _____

See Section III for differential diagnosis, appropriate follow-up, and brief case review.

A 30-year-old female is seen in the office complaining of pain in her right hand for the past 6 months.

She complains that the pain has been worsening gradually. She describes the pain as a burning type of pain which affects all of the fingers in her right hand with the exception of her little finger. The pain travels up her arm almost to the shoulder. She states that the pain is bad during the day and worse at night, occasionally waking her up. She has also noticed that she has pain in other areas which include her shoulders, neck, and back. The pain in these areas feels different from the pain in her hand and is not as severe. She has never experienced morning stiffness. She has been healthy in the past and has never been hospitalized for any reason. She lives with her husband and their two children. She is employed as a typist in a hospital. She denies the use of alcohol and cigarettes.

Patient History Checklist

- ☐ Patient's name
- ☐ Patient's age
- ☐ Patient's address
- ☐ Patient's occupation
- ☐ Patient's presenting complaint
- ☐ Absence/presence of pain
- ☐ History of the pain
  - ☐ Site
  - ☐ Onset
  - ☐ Duration
  - ☐ Intensity
  - ☐ Radiation
  - ☐ Character
  - ☐ Exacerbating factors

   ☐ Relieving factors
   ☐ Medications used to relieve symptoms
☐ Presence of pain on movement
☐ Swelling of the affected area
☐ Redness of the affected area
☐ Presence of nausea/vomiting
☐ Presence of fatigue
☐ Presence of fever
☐ Previous episodes of symptoms
☐ History of trauma
☐ History of recent surgery
☐ History of repetitive activities—occupation, sports, recreational
☐ Medical history
☐ Hospital admissions
☐ Surgical history
☐ Medications
☐ Last menstrual period
☐ Family history
   ☐ Heart disease
   ☐ Diabetes
   ☐ Thyroid disease
   ☐ Cancer
   ☐ Others
☐ Social history
   ☐ Smoking
   ☐ Alcohol
   ☐ Other drug use

Differential Diagnosis

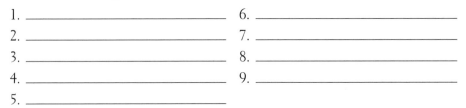

1. _____   6. _____
2. _____   7. _____
3. _____   8. _____
4. _____   9. _____
5. _____

Physical Examination Checklist

- ☐ Overall assessment—pay particular attention to signs of endocrine disease (acromegaly, hypothyroidism, diabetes mellitus)
- ☐ Vitals
  - ☐ Temperature
  - ☐ Pulse
  - ☐ Blood pressure
  - ☐ Respirations
- ☐ Examine the extremities (bilaterally)
  - ☐ Inspect upper extremities
    - ☐ Symmetry
    - ☐ Deformities
    - ☐ Muscle wasting
    - ☐ Swellings
    - ☐ Areas of erythema
    - ☐ Active range of motion
  - ☐ Palpate upper extremities
    - ☐ Temperature
    - ☐ Tenderness
    - ☐ Masses
- ☐ Assess passive range of motion
- ☐ Assess mobility of the wrist joints
- ☐ Assess mobility of the finger joints
- ☐ Check for pain and crude touch in the hands
- ☐ Check for light touch in the hands
- ☐ Perform Phalen's test
- ☐ Check for Tinel's sign
- ☐ Examine the cervical spine
  - ☐ Symmetry
  - ☐ Deformities
  - ☐ Swelling
  - ☐ Redness
  - ☐ Active range of motion
- ☐ Palpate
  - ☐ Temperature
  - ☐ Tenderness
  - ☐ Masses

☐ Check reflexes
   ☐ Biceps
   ☐ Triceps
   ☐ Brachioradialis

Physical Examination Findings

General: 30-year-old female, no acute distress

Vitals:

   Pulse—82/minute   Temperature—97.9°F

   BP—118/76 mm Hg   Respirations—14/minute

Upper extremities:

   Symmetrical, no muscle atrophy noted

   No scarring, deformities, swellings, or areas of erythema

   Normal active range of motion bilaterally

   Temperature equal bilaterally

   No tenderness to palpation noted

   No masses appreciated

   Decreased sensation to pain and light touch in the distribution of the median nerve on the right

   Phalen's test positive on the right

   Tinel's sign present on the right

Cervical spine:

   No deformities, swelling, or redness

   Normal active range of motion

   No areas of increased temperature appreciated

   No masses appreciated

   No tenderness to palpation

Deep tendon reflexes intact

Differential Diagnosis

1. _____   3. _____
2. _____   4. _____

Follow-Up

1. _____   4. _____
2. _____   5. _____
3. _____

See Section III for differential diagnosis, appropriate follow-up, and brief case review.

A 43-year-old male is seen in the clinic for follow-up of his recent foot pain.

He is very concerned about a pain that he has recently experienced in his foot. He states that the pain started approximately 10 days ago while he was visiting family in New York. The pain came on very suddenly overnight, localized to his right big toe. It was so severe that he could not walk, he could only bear weight on his heel. The toe was also warm to the touch and appeared very red. He states that at the time he also felt slightly feverish and nauseated. He was seen in the emergency room in New York at the time of onset and an X-ray was done which did not reveal any abnormalities. The pain and swelling was severe for approximately 1 week and then resolved. He noticed that the skin over his big toe peeled off. He has had no further symptoms since that time. He had a similar episode 2 years ago and has come to the clinic to see if he can find out what is going on and if the source of these episodes of pain can be determined.

Patient History Checklist

- ☐ Patient's name
- ☐ Patient's age
- ☐ Patient's address
- ☐ Patient's occupation
- ☐ Patient's presenting complaint
- ☐ Absence/presence of pain
- ☐ History of the pain
  - ☐ Site
  - ☐ Onset
  - ☐ Duration
  - ☐ Intensity
  - ☐ Radiation
  - ☐ Character
  - ☐ Exacerbating factors

- ☐ Relieving factors
- ☐ Medications used to relieve symptoms
- ☐ Presence of pain on movement
- ☐ Swelling of the affected area
- ☐ Redness of the affected area
- ☐ Presence of nausea/vomiting
- ☐ Presence of fatigue
- ☐ Presence of fever
- ☐ Presence of morning stiffness
- ☐ Previous episodes of symptoms
- ☐ History of trauma
- ☐ History of recent surgery
- ☐ Use of diuretics
- ☐ History of alcoholic binge drinking
- ☐ Diet (particularly high protein diet)
- ☐ History of unusual exercise
- ☐ History of exposure to toxic heavy metals, particularly lead
- ☐ Medical history
- ☐ Hospital admissions
- ☐ Surgical history
- ☐ Medications
- ☐ Family history
  - ☐ Gout
  - ☐ Heart disease
  - ☐ Diabetes
  - ☐ Thyroid disease
  - ☐ Cancer
  - ☐ Others
- ☐ Social history
  - ☐ Smoking
  - ☐ Alcohol
  - ☐ Other drug use

Differential Diagnosis

1. _____   6. _____
2. _____   7. _____
3. _____   8. _____
4. _____   9. _____
5. _____

Physical Examination Checklist

☐ Overall assessment
☐ Vitals
   ☐ Temperature
   ☐ Pulse
   ☐ Blood pressure
   ☐ Respirations
☐ Observe patients gait
☐ Examine the extremities
   ☐ Inspect lower extremities
      ☐ Symmetry
      ☐ Deformities
      ☐ Swellings
      ☐ Areas of erythema
   ☐ Palpate lower extremities
      ☐ Temperature
      ☐ Tenderness
      ☐ Masses
   ☐ Assess mobility of hip joints
   ☐ Assess mobility of knee joints
   ☐ Assess mobility of ankle joints
   ☐ Assess mobility of the foot joints
   ☐ Perform a full cardiovascular examination, if time permits

Physical Examination Findings

General: 44-year-old male, no acute distress
Vitals:

Pulse — 80/minute	Temperature — 97.4°F
BP — 112/76 mm Hg	Respirations — 14/minute

No abnormal gait noted
Lower extremities:

Symmetrical

No deformities, ecchymosis, or scars noted

No erythema

Temperature equal bilaterally

No masses appreciated

Full active range of motion at hips, knees, ankles, and foot joints

Differential Diagnosis

1. _____   3. _____
2. _____   4. _____

Follow-Up

1. _____   4. _____
2. _____   5. _____
3. _____

See Section III for differential diagnosis, appropriate follow-up, and brief case review.

CASE 21

A 34-year-old female presents concerning her inability to conceive.

The patient reports that she and her husband have been trying to conceive a child for the past few years. She previously took the birth control pill, but stopped using it 6 years ago. Since that time she and her husband have not used any form of contraceptive. Her inability to conceive was first investigated a few years ago when she complained of some leaking from her breasts. She has only had two periods since stopping the pill 6 years ago. Her last period was 4 months ago. She has been treated in the past with the fertility drug clomid without results and is currently taking parlodel but still has had no success. She has no significant medical history. She states that she enjoys intercourse and she and her husband have intercourse three to four times a week. She is requesting some help as her husband desperately wants to have a child and she has begun to feel very depressed about the whole situation.

Patient History Checklist

- ☐ Patient's name
- ☐ Patient's age
- ☐ Patient's address
- ☐ Patient's occupation
- ☐ Patient's presenting complaint
- ☐ Sexual history
  - ☐ Age of menarche
  - ☐ Frequency of periods
  - ☐ Last menstrual period
  - ☐ Duration of periods
  - ☐ Presence of dysmenorrhea
  - ☐ Frequency of sexual intercourse
  - ☐ Interest in sexual intercourse
  - ☐ History of sexually transmitted diseases

- ☐ Presence of vaginal discharge
- ☐ Presence of dyspareunia
- ☐ Number of pregnancies/outcomes of pregnancies
- ☐ Number of abortions
- ☐ Reasons for abortions
- ☐ Presence of excess facial hair
- ☐ Presence of weight loss/gain
- ☐ Amount of weight loss/weight gain
- ☐ Time period of weight loss/weight gain
- ☐ Presence of nipple discharge
- ☐ Partner's details
  - ☐ Age
  - ☐ Occupation
  - ☐ History of sexually transmitted diseases
  - ☐ Number of children, if any
  - ☐ Ability to achieve vaginal penetration
  - ☐ Frequency of ejaculation
- ☐ Medical history
- ☐ Hospital admissions
- ☐ Surgical history
- ☐ Medications
- ☐ Family history
  - ☐ Siblings with children
  - ☐ Depression
  - ☐ Psychiatric illnesses
  - ☐ Heart disease
  - ☐ Diabetes
  - ☐ Thyroid disease
  - ☐ Cancer
  - ☐ Others
- ☐ Social history
  - ☐ Smoking
  - ☐ Alcohol
  - ☐ Other drug use
  - ☐ Family situation
  - ☐ Feelings of anxiety
  - ☐ Exercise

Differential Diagnosis

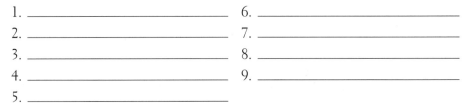

1. _____   6. _____
2. _____   7. _____
3. _____   8. _____
4. _____   9. _____
5. _____

Physical Examination Checklist

- ☐ Overall assessment
- ☐ Vitals
  - ☐ Temperature
  - ☐ Pulse
  - ☐ Blood pressure
  - ☐ Respirations
- ☐ Observe for evidence of endocrine disorder
- ☐ Assess hair distribution
- ☐ Examine the abdomen
  - ☐ Inspect
  - ☐ Auscultate
  - ☐ Light palpation
  - ☐ Deep palpation
  - ☐ Assess for organomegaly (palpation and percussion)
  - ☐ Assess for pelvic abdominal masses
- ☐ Indicate to the patient that you would like to perform a breast examination and a pelvic examination, but will not do so during this examination

Physical Examination Findings

General: 34-year-old female, no acute distress

Vitals:

Pulse—78/minute   Temperature—98.8°F

BP—115/70 mm Hg   Respirations—12/minute

Normal female hair distribution, no facial hair noted

Abdomen:

    No ecchymosis visible

    No visible masses

    No striae noted

    No visible peristalsis

    Normal female hair distribution

    Bowel sounds present in all quadrants

    No bruits heard

    No friction rubs over the spleen or liver

    No tenderness to palpation

    No hepatosplenomegaly

Differential Diagnosis

1. _____   3. _____

2. _____   4. _____

Follow-Up

1. _____   4. _____

2. _____   5. _____

3. _____

See Section III for differential diagnosis, appropriate follow-up, and brief case review.

CASE 22

A 25-year-old male is seen in the outpatient clinic complaining of diarrhea.

The patient states that the diarrhea started approximately 2 weeks ago and is so severe that it is interfering with his job. He has been having diarrhea 8–10 times a day. He complains of some mild abdominal discomfort associated with the diarrhea. There is no blood or mucus in the stool. His appetite has been poor and he has been having some difficulty sleeping. When questioned about his medical history he tells the physician that he is HIV positive. He was first tested 3 years ago when he had an outbreak of shingles. He has had two episodes of pneumonia; however, he cannot remember the name of the organism involved. He is currently taking retrovir, combivir, and bactrim.

Patient History Checklist

☐ Patient's name
☐ Patient's age
☐ Patient's address
☐ Patient's occupation
☐ Patient's presenting complaint
☐ Changes in bowel movements
☐ Frequency of bowel movements
☐ Presence of blood/mucus in the stool
☐ Contacts with diarrhea
☐ Recent travel history
☐ Ill contacts
☐ Change in diet
☐ Changes in appetite (increased/decreased)
☐ Presence of weight loss/gain
☐ Amount of weight loss/weight gain
☐ Time period of weight loss/weight gain
☐ Presence of pain

- ☐ History of the pain
    - ☐ Site
    - ☐ Onset
    - ☐ Duration
    - ☐ Intensity
    - ☐ Radiation
    - ☐ Character
    - ☐ Exacerbating factors
    - ☐ Relieving factors
- ☐ Medical history
- ☐ AIDS-associated illnesses, past/present
- ☐ Hospital admissions
- ☐ Surgical history
- ☐ Current medications
- ☐ Sexual history
    - ☐ Sexual orientation
    - ☐ Sexual activity
    - ☐ History of sexually transmitted diseases
    - ☐ Practice of safe sex
    - ☐ Partners' HIV status
    - ☐ Knowledge of AIDS transmission and the natural progression of the disease
- ☐ Family history
    - ☐ Heart disease
    - ☐ Diabetes
    - ☐ Thyroid disease
    - ☐ Cancer
    - ☐ Others
- ☐ Social history
    - ☐ Smoking
    - ☐ Alcohol
    - ☐ Other drug use (in particular, injectable drugs)

Differential Diagnosis

1. _____   6. _____
2. _____   7. _____
3. _____   8. _____
4. _____   9. _____
5. _____

Physical Examination Checklist

- ☐ Overall assessment
- ☐ Vitals
  - ☐ Temperature—assess for fever
  - ☐ Pulse—assess for tachycardia
  - ☐ Blood pressure
  - ☐ Respirations
- ☐ Examine the eyes
  - ☐ Assess for conjunctival pallor
- ☐ Examine the mouth
  - ☐ Assess for signs of nutritional deficiencies
  - ☐ Assess for signs of dehydration
  - ☐ Assess for signs of infection
- ☐ Examine the abdomen
  - ☐ Inspect
  - ☐ Auscultate
  - ☐ Light palpation
  - ☐ Deep palpation
  - ☐ Assess for organomegaly (palpation and percussion)
  - ☐ Assess for muscular rigidity
  - ☐ Assess for rebound tenderness
- ☐ Perform a complete physical examination if time permits to assess for other features of AIDS

Physical Examination Findings

General: 25-year-old male, uncomfortable appearing
Vitals:

    Pulse—92/minute   Temperature—97.9°F

    BP—114/80 mm Hg   Respirations—14/minute

HEENT:

    Eyes—No conjunctival pallor noted

    Mouth

        No crackes/fissures noted

        No pallor

        Mucous membranes moist

        No candida noted

        No dental caries noted

Abdomen:

    No ecchymosis visible

    No visible masses

    No striae noted

    No visible peristalsis

    Bowel sounds present in all quadrants

    No bruits heard

    No friction rubs over the spleen or liver

    No tenderness to palpation

    No hepatosplenomegaly

    No rebound tenderness

Differential Diagnosis

1. _____   3. _____

2. _____   4. _____

Follow-Up

1. _____   4. _____

2. _____   5. _____

3. _____

See Section III for differential diagnosis, appropriate follow-up, and brief case review.

A 29-year-old male is seen in the clinic complaining of discomfort while urinating.

The patient complains that is has been painful to urinate for the past 3 days. He finds that the pain occurs while he is passing urine and subsides following the passage of urine. He has not experienced any abdominal pain. He has also noticed that he has a discharge from his penis. The discharge is greenish in color and mostly present in the morning. He has had the discharge for the past 3 days. He has not noticed any fever associated with these symptoms. He has been tested for sexually transmitted diseases in the past and the only thing that he is aware that he has is herpes. He was diagnosed with herpes 5 years ago. He currently has about one outbreak per year. He is in a monogamous relationship with his same sex partner. They are both tested annually for HIV and are both negative.

Patient History Checklist

- ☐ Patient's name
- ☐ Patient's age
- ☐ Patient's address
- ☐ Patient's occupation
- ☐ Patient's presenting complaint
- ☐ Frequency of micturition
- ☐ Presence of dysuria
- ☐ Presence of nocturia
- ☐ Presence of hematuria
- ☐ Previous episodes of similar symptoms
- ☐ Absence/presence of abdominal pain
- ☐ Presence of discharge from penis
- ☐ Appearance of discharge
- ☐ Presence of fever
- ☐ Sexual history

    ☐ Number of sexual partners
    ☐ History of sexually transmitted diseases
    ☐ Use of condoms
    ☐ HIV status
☐ Changes in bowel movements
☐ Changes in appetite (increased/decreased)
☐ Medical history
☐ Hospital admissions
☐ Surgical history
☐ Medications
☐ Family history
    ☐ Kidney disease
    ☐ Heart disease
    ☐ Diabetes
    ☐ Thyroid disease
    ☐ Cancer
    ☐ Others
☐ Social history
    ☐ Smoking
    ☐ Alcohol
    ☐ Other drug use

Differential Diagnosis

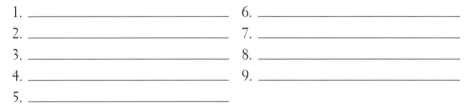

1. _____   6. _____
2. _____   7. _____
3. _____   8. _____
4. _____   9. _____
5. _____

Physical Examination Checklist

☐ Overall assessment
☐ Vitals
    ☐ Temperature—assess for fever
    ☐ Pulse—assess for tachycardia

- ☐ Blood pressure
- ☐ Respirations
☐ Examine the abdomen
  - ☐ Inspect
  - ☐ Auscultate
  - ☐ Light palpation
  - ☐ Deep palpation
  - ☐ Assess for organomegaly (palpation and percussion)
  - ☐ Assess for CVA tenderness
  - ☐ Assess for muscular rigidity
  - ☐ Assess for referred rebound tenderness
  - ☐ Assess for rebound tenderness
☐ Indicate to the patient that you would like to examine his genitalia, but will not do so during this examination

Physical Examination Findings

General: 29-year-old male, no acute distress

Vitals:

Pulse—86/minute	Temperature—98.3°F
BP—126/88 mm Hg	Respirations—14/minute

Abdomen:

No ecchymosis visible

No visible masses

No striae noted

No visible peristalsis

Bowel sounds present in all quadrants

No bruits heard

No friction rubs over the spleen or liver

No tenderness to palpation noted

No hepatosplenomegaly

No CVA tenderness

No referred rebound tenderness noted

No rebound tenderness

Differential Diagnosis

1. _____   3. _____

2. _____   4. _____

Follow-Up

1. _____   4. _____

2. _____   5. _____

3. _____

See Section III for differential diagnosis, appropriate follow-up, and brief case review.

CASE 24

A 23-year-old male is brought to the clinic following an injury during a soccer game. He is complaining of left knee pain.

The patient reports that during the game, he and another player collided with each other. The other player ran into his left side. He immediately fell to the ground and has been experiencing severe knee pain since that time. He describes the pain as an aching and throbbing pain and as an 8 on a scale of 1–10, with 10 being the most severe pain. He has been playing soccer for the past 10 years. He has never been injured while playing in the past with the exception of the occasional bruise or abrasion. He has not had any previous injury to his left knee. His medical history is unremarkable. He has never been hospitalized and has never had any surgeries. There is no significant family history.

Patient History Checklist

- ☐ Patient's name
- ☐ Patient's age
- ☐ Patient's address
- ☐ Patient's occupation
- ☐ Patient's presenting complaint
- ☐ Absence/presence of pain
- ☐ History of the pain
  - ☐ Site
  - ☐ Onset
  - ☐ Duration
  - ☐ Intensity
  - ☐ Radiation
  - ☐ Character
  - ☐ Exacerbating factors
  - ☐ Relieving factors
  - ☐ Medications used to relieve symptoms

☐ Mechanism of injury
☐ Presence of pain on movement
☐ Swelling of the affected area
☐ Redness of the affected area
☐ Ability to bear weight
☐ Previous episodes of symptoms
☐ History of trauma
☐ History of recent surgery
☐ Medical history
☐ Hospital admissions
☐ Surgical history
☐ Medications
☐ Family history
   ☐ Heart disease
   ☐ Diabetes
   ☐ Thyroid disease
   ☐ Cancer
   ☐ Others
☐ Social history
   ☐ Smoking
   ☐ Alcohol
   ☐ Other drug use

Differential Diagnosis

1. _____   6. _____
2. _____   7. _____
3. _____   8. _____
4. _____   9. _____
5. _____

Physical Examination Checklist

☐ Overall assessment
☐ Vitals
   ☐ Temperature

- ☐ Pulse
- ☐ Blood pressure
- ☐ Respirations
- ☐ Observe patients gait
- ☐ Examine the extremities
  - ☐ Inspect lower extremities
    - ☐ Symmetry
    - ☐ Deformities
    - ☐ Swellings
    - ☐ Areas of erythema
  - ☐ Palpate lower extremities
    - ☐ Temperature
    - ☐ Tenderness
    - ☐ Masses
- ☐ Assess mobility of hip joints
- ☐ Assess mobility of knee joints
- ☐ Assess mobility of ankle joints
- ☐ Assess mobility of the foot joints
- ☐ Bulge sign
- ☐ Ballottement
- ☐ Drawer sign
- ☐ Assessment of collateral ligaments
- ☐ McMurray's test
- ☐ Perform a full physical examination, if time permits, looking for any other signs of trauma or injury

Physical Examination Findings

General: 23-year-old male, no acute distress

Vitals:

Pulse—78/minute	Temperature—97.4°F
BP—122/78 mm Hg	Respirations—12/minute

Patient noted to be having difficulty ambulating. Unable to weight bear on left leg.

Lower extremities:

   Asymmetrical

   No deformities, ecchymosis, or scars noted

   Mild erythema of left knee noted

   Mild swelling of left knee noted

   Left knee warm on palpation

   No masses appreciated

   Full active range of motion at hips, ankles, and foot joints

   Limited range of motion of left knee due to pain

   Bulge test negative

   Ballottment negative

   McMurrays test negative

   Assessment of lateral collateral ligament normal

   Assessment of medial collateral ligament abnormal—patient experienc-
      ing a great deal of pain during examination. Some movement of the
      joint appreciated

   Drawer sign negative

Differential Diagnosis

1. _____   3. _____
2. _____   4. _____

Follow-Up

1. _____   4. _____
2. _____   5. _____
3. _____

See Section III for differential diagnosis, appropriate follow-up, and brief case
review.

CASE 25

A 59-year-old male has been brought to the emergency room by the police after being found unresponsive in the street.

Upon arrival, the patient started to regain consciousness and a strong odor of alcohol was detected on his breath. Several hours later the patient is awake, alert, and oriented. When questioned carefully, the patient admits that he drinks a bottle of vodka a day along with several beers. He is currently living in a half way house, which houses 14 other people. He is unemployed. He has not been feeling well for the past 3 months. He has been experiencing intermittent fevers, chills, and a significant amount of weight loss. He reports that he has been experiencing night sweats and often has to get up in the night to dry off. He developed a cough approximately 3–4 months ago, which was associated with some chest pain. He has often seen blood in his sputum but has just assumed that this was associated with his cigarette smoking and would resolve if he gave up smoking. He currently smokes 1 pack of cigarettes per day and has done so for the past 35 years.

Patient History Checklist

☐ Patient's name
☐ Patient's age
☐ Patient's address
☐ Patient's occupation
☐ Patient's presenting complaint
☐ Duration of symptoms
☐ Presence of cough (productive/nonproductive)
☐ Appearance of the sputum
☐ Presence of blood in the sputum
☐ Shortness of breath
☐ Presence of fever
☐ History of weight loss

- ☐ Amount of weight loss
- ☐ Time period of weight loss
- ☐ Presence of night sweats
- ☐ Presence of chest pain
- ☐ History of the pain
    - ☐ Site
    - ☐ Onset
    - ☐ Duration
    - ☐ Intensity
    - ☐ Radiation
    - ☐ Character
    - ☐ Exacerbating factors
    - ☐ Relieving factors
- ☐ Ill contacts
- ☐ Nausea/ vomiting/diarrhea
- ☐ Presence of rhinorrhea
- ☐ History of delirium tremens
- ☐ History of opportunistic infections (typical of AIDS)
- ☐ Medical history
- ☐ Hospital admissions
- ☐ Surgical history
- ☐ Medications
- ☐ Family history
    - ☐ Cancer
    - ☐ Heart disease
    - ☐ Diabetes
    - ☐ Thyroid disease
    - ☐ Asthma/allergies
    - ☐ Others
- ☐ Social history
    - ☐ Smoking
    - ☐ Alcohol (CAGE questions)
    - ☐ Other drug use
    - ☐ Living situation (crowded conditions)

Differential Diagnosis

1. _____   6. _____

2. _____   7. _____

3. _____   8. _____

4. _____   9. _____

5. _____

Physical Examination Checklist

☐ Overall assessment
☐ Vitals
   ☐ Temperature—assess for fever
   ☐ Pulse—assess for tachycardia
   ☐ Blood pressure
   ☐ Respirations—assess for tachypnea
☐ Examine the face
   ☐ Assess mucus membranes for the presence of cyanosis
☐ Examine the mouth
   ☐ Assess for signs of nutritional deficiencies
   ☐ Assess for signs of dehydration
   ☐ Assess for signs of infection
☐ Examine the neck
   ☐ Assess for lymphadenopathy
   ☐ Assess for use of accessory muscles
   ☐ Assess the position of the trachea
☐ Examine the extremities
   ☐ Assess for clubbing
   ☐ Assess for cyanosis
☐ Respiratory system—examine the thorax
   ☐ Inspect
      ☐ Size
      ☐ Shape
      ☐ Symmetry
      ☐ Movement
      ☐ Deformities of the ribs

    ☐ Deformities of the spine
    ☐ Scars
  ☐ Palpate
    ☐ Tenderness
    ☐ Excursion
    ☐ Tactile fremitus
    ☐ Chest dimensions
    ☐ Position of the diaphragm
  ☐ Percuss
    ☐ All areas comparing side to side
    ☐ Diaphragm excursion (left)
    ☐ Diaphragm excursion (right)
  ☐ Auscultate
    ☐ All areas comparing side to side
    ☐ Breath sounds
    ☐ Vocal resonance
    ☐ Whispering pectoriloquy
    ☐ Aegophony
☐ Examine the abdomen
  ☐ General examination for signs of hepatic failure
  ☐ Inspect
  ☐ Auscultate
  ☐ Light palpation
  ☐ Deep palpation
  ☐ Assess for organomegaly (palpation and percussion)
  ☐ Assess for fluid wave
  ☐ Assess for shifting dullness

Physical Examination Findings

General: 59-year-old male. Patient appearing lethargic. Strong odor of alcohol detectable on his breath.

Vitals:

Pulse—102/minute	Temperature—101.8°F
BP—108/68 mm Hg	Respirations—22/minute

HEENT:

Mouth—Mucous membranes dry; No cyanosis noted

Extremities: No clubbing or cyanosis noted

Neck:

No lymphadenopathy

No use of accessory muscles of respirations noted

Trachea midline

Respiratory system:

Thorax normal size and shape

No asymmetry noted

No scars or deformities noted

No tenderness to palpation

Excursion equal bilaterally

Tactile fremitus equal bilaterally

No increased anteroposterior diameter

Dull to percussion at right base

Level of the diaphragms equal bilaterally

Breath sounds decreased at right base

No wheezing noted

No vocal resonance noted

No whispering pectoriloquy noted

No aegophony noted

Abdomen:

No ecchymosis visible

No visible masses

No striae noted

No visible peristalsis

Bowel sounds present in all quadrants

No bruits heard

No friction rubs over the spleen or liver

Mild tenderness to palpation in pelvic region

No hepatosplenomegaly
No fluid wave noted
No shifting dullness noted

Differential Diagnosis

1. _____   3. _____
2. _____   4. _____

Follow-Up

1. _____   4. _____
2. _____   5. _____
3. _____

See Section III for differential diagnosis, appropriate follow-up, and brief case review.

CASE 26

A 32-year-old female is seen by her primary care physician. She states that she has been having pain in her hands and knees for the past 6 months.

She reports that the first time that she experienced the symptoms was in the morning. She states that at the onset of her symptoms she felt very stiff in the mornings for approximately 30 minutes and then the stiffness would resolve and not reappear again until the next morning. She complains that the symptoms have been getting progressively worse over the past 6 months and she is now having difficulty with her normal daily activities. She still experiences a great deal of stiffness in the morning, but now the stiffness does not resolve until after lunch. She also has noticed that she has been feeling stiff in the evenings while watching television. She has been very fatigued over the past 6 months and finds that she is having difficulty doing basic household chores as she now goes to bed just after dinner in the evenings. She has had to miss quite a few days of work due to the severity of her symptoms. She works as a personal secretary and on occasion has had difficulty taking shorthand and typing. She lives alone. She denies the use of cigarettes and alcohol. Her medical history is unremarkable.

Patient History Checklist

- ☐ Patient's name
- ☐ Patient's age
- ☐ Patient's address
- ☐ Patient's occupation
- ☐ Patient's presenting complaint
- ☐ Absence/presence of pain
- ☐ History of the pain
  - ☐ Site
  - ☐ Onset
  - ☐ Duration
  - ☐ Intensity

- ☐ Radiation
- ☐ Character
- ☐ Exacerbating factors
- ☐ Relieving factors
- ☐ Medications used to relieve symptoms
☐ Presence of pain on movement
☐ Swelling of the affected area
☐ Redness of the affected area
☐ Presence of Raynaud's phenomenon
☐ Presence of nausea/vomiting
☐ Presence of fatigue
☐ Presence of fever
☐ Presence of irritation and/or redness of the eyes
☐ Absence of morning stiffness
☐ Previous episodes of symptoms
☐ History of trauma
☐ History of recent surgery
☐ Frequency of micturition
☐ Presence of dysuria
☐ Use of diuretics
☐ History of alcoholic binge drinking
☐ History of unusual exercise
☐ Medical history
☐ Hospital admissions
☐ Surgical history
☐ Medications
☐ Family history
- ☐ Rheumatoid arthritis
- ☐ Heart disease
- ☐ Diabetes
- ☐ Thyroid disease
- ☐ Cancer
- ☐ Others
☐ Social history
- ☐ Smoking
- ☐ Alcohol
- ☐ Other drug use

Differential Diagnosis

1. _____   6. _____
2. _____   7. _____
3. _____   8. _____
4. _____   9. _____
5. _____

Physical Examination Checklist

- ☐ Overall assessment
- ☐ Vitals
  - ☐ Temperature
  - ☐ Pulse
  - ☐ Blood pressure
  - ☐ Respirations
- ☐ Observe patient's gait
- ☐ Examine the extremities (bilaterally)
  - ☐ Inspect upper extremities
    - ☐ Symmetry
    - ☐ Deformities
    - ☐ Swellings
    - ☐ Areas of erythema
  - ☐ Palpate upper extremities
    - ☐ Temperature
    - ☐ Tenderness
    - ☐ Masses
  - ☐ Inspect lower extremities
    - ☐ Symmetry
    - ☐ Deformities
    - ☐ Swellings
    - ☐ Areas of erythema
  - ☐ Palpate lower extremities
    - ☐ Temperature
    - ☐ Tenderness
    - ☐ Masses

☐ Assess mobility of hip joints
☐ Assess mobility of knee joints
☐ Assess mobility of ankle joints
☐ Assess mobility of the finger joints
☐ Assess mobility of the foot joints
☐ Check all reflexes
    ☐ Abdominal
    ☐ Plantar
    ☐ Biceps
    ☐ Triceps
    ☐ Brachioradialis
    ☐ Quadriceps
    ☐ Knee
    ☐ Ankle
☐ Examine the eyes, paying particular attention to any inflammation of the conjunctiva or the iris

Physical Examination Findings

General: 32-year-old female, uncomfortable appearing

Vitals:

    Pulse—76/minute   Temperature—97.3°F

    BP—118/68 mm Hg   Respirations—12/minute

    No abnormal gait observed

Upper extremities:

    Symmetrical

    No ecchymosis, erythema, swellings, or deformities noted

    Marked tenderness to palpation of wrist and finger joints

    Temperature equal bilaterally

Lower extremities:

    Symmetrical

    No ecchymosis, erythema, swellings, or deformities noted

    Mild tenderness to palpation of ankle joints

    Temperature equal bilaterally

Limited range of motion of finger, wrist, and ankle joints
Full active range of motion at hips, and knees
Deep tendon reflexes intact
Abdominal reflex present
Plantar reflex down going

Differential Diagnosis

1. _____   3. _____
2. _____   4. _____

Follow-Up

1. _____   4. _____
2. _____   5. _____
3. _____

See Section III for differential diagnosis, appropriate follow-up, and brief case review.

CASE 27

The father of a 5-year-old boy comes to the outpatient clinic. He states that his son is still wetting the bed at night.

He has not brought his son with him to the visit for fear that it would only upset the child and make matters worse. He states that his son has been out of diapers during the day since the age of 2. He wore a diaper to bed until the age of 4. His son tends to wet the bed approximately three to four times per week. He is very concerned that this is going to continue to be a problem and that his son may never outgrow this. He notices that his son does not seem to wake up to go to the bathroom. He has tried to limit his son's fluid intake in the evening but this does not seem to have any effect. His son has never had any medical problems and seems to be happy with the school that he attends. He is an only child.

Patient History Checklist

- ☐ Patient's name
- ☐ Patient's age
- ☐ Patient's address
- ☐ Patient's presenting complaint
- ☐ Episodes of enuresis per week
- ☐ Episodes of incontinence of urine during the day
- ☐ Episodes of incontinence to feces
- ☐ Stress at home
- ☐ Stress at school
- ☐ Episodes of tearfulness
- ☐ Frequency of micturition
- ☐ Presence of dysuria
- ☐ Presence of hematuria
- ☐ Changes in appetite
- ☐ Presence of weight loss/gain

☐ Amount of weight loss/weight gain
☐ Time period of weight loss/weight gain
☐ Medical history
☐ Birth history
    ☐ Weeks of gestation at delivery
    ☐ Complications during the pregnancy
    ☐ Duration of labor
    ☐ Complications during delivery
    ☐ Immunizations up to date
☐ Family history of diseases (mother, father, and siblings)
    ☐ Enuresis
    ☐ Psychiatric disorders
    ☐ Heart disease
    ☐ Diabetes
    ☐ Thyroid disease
    ☐ Sickle-cell disease
☐ Social history
    ☐ Living situation
    ☐ Pets in the home
    ☐ Smoking in the home

Differential Diagnosis

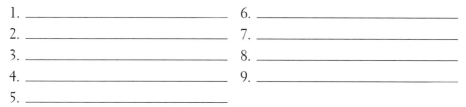

1. _____   6. _____
2. _____   7. _____
3. _____   8. _____
4. _____   9. _____
5. _____

Physical Examination Checklist

Advise the father to return to the clinic with his son for a full assessment.

Follow-Up

1. _____   4. _____

2. _____   5. _____

3. _____

See Section III for differential diagnosis, appropriate follow-up, and brief case review.

CASE 28

A 69-year-old man is seen in the outpatient department. He complains of feeling tired. He also complains that he is experiencing aches and pains throughout his body.

The patient reports that he has been feeling generally unwell since the death of his wife. He has experienced migrating aches and pains in all of his limbs. He does not report that there is any specific time of day that his symptoms are worse. He has been feeling lethargic and finds that he is sleeping much more than usual. He has not noticed any swelling of any joints or any redness of any joints and has not had a fever. His wife passed away very suddenly 2 weeks ago. He and his wife were married for 42 years and have one son together. The son lives in Canada and was in attendance at his mother's funeral, but stayed only for a couple of days before he had to return home to Canada. The patient becomes tearful during the interview as he talks about his wife. He states that his wife was his best friend and since her passing he has been very lonely and unsure how to spend his days. He is retired. His only real hobby is playing cards, which he used to do with his wife and their friends twice a week. Since his wife passed away he does not feel that he would be welcomed by the group with which they used to play and feels that he would be out of place if he were to attend without his wife. When questioned about the symptoms that brought him to the office he is vague and does not give much detail.

Patient History Checklist

☐ Patient's name
☐ Patient's age
☐ Patient's address
☐ Patient's occupation
☐ Patient's presenting complaint
☐ Duration of symptoms
☐ Presence of fatigue

- ☐ Presence of irritability
- ☐ Difficulty concentrating
- ☐ Difficulty sleeping
- ☐ Presence of early morning waking
- ☐ Loss of appetite
- ☐ Presence of weight loss/gain
- ☐ Amount of weight loss/weight gain
- ☐ Time period of weight loss/weight gain
- ☐ Ability to function at home
- ☐ Presence of support system
- ☐ Loss of interest in hobbies
- ☐ Tearfulness
- ☐ Feelings of worthlessness
- ☐ Suicidal ideation
  - ☐ Suicide plan
  - ☐ Previous suicide attempts
- ☐ History of the pain
  - ☐ Site
  - ☐ Onset
  - ☐ Duration
  - ☐ Intensity
  - ☐ Radiation
  - ☐ Character
  - ☐ Exacerbating factors
  - ☐ Relieving factors
  - ☐ Medications used to relieve symptoms
- ☐ Presence of pain on movement
- ☐ Swelling of the affected area
- ☐ Redness of the affected area
- ☐ Presence of Raynaud's phenomenon
- ☐ Presence of nausea/vomiting
- ☐ Presence of fever
- ☐ Presence of irritation and/or redness of the eyes
- ☐ Absence of morning stiffness
- ☐ Previous episodes of symptoms
- ☐ History of trauma
- ☐ Medical history
- ☐ Hospital admissions

☐ Surgical history
☐ Medications
☐ Family history
    ☐ Depression
    ☐ Psychiatric illnesses
    ☐ Heart disease
    ☐ Diabetes
    ☐ Thyroid disease
    ☐ Cancer
    ☐ Others
☐ Social history
    ☐ Smoking
    ☐ Alcohol
    ☐ Other drug use
    ☐ Family situation

Differential Diagnosis

1. _____   6. _____
2. _____   7. _____
3. _____   8. _____
4. _____   9. _____
5. _____

Physical Examination Checklist

If time permits, perform an examination of the musculoskeletal system.

Follow-Up

1. _____   4. _____
2. _____   5. _____
3. _____

See Section III for differential diagnosis, appropriate follow-up, and brief case review.

CASE 29

A 45-year-old male is seen in the clinic for follow-up of his hypertension.

The patient was initially found to be hypertensive 5 years ago. He currently takes only one medication for control of his blood pressure. His blood pressure has been well controlled since the time of diagnosis and the patient is very compliant with both medication and regular checkups. He has no other significant medical history. He is mildly obese, but has maintained a steady weight since the time of his diagnosis. He eats a healthy diet and is aware of his salt intake. He was previously a smoker, but quit smoking at the time of his diagnosis and has remained a nonsmoker since that time. He lives at home with his wife and their three children. His family history is significant for thyroid disease and heart disease.

Patient History Checklist

☐ Patient's name
☐ Patient's age
☐ Patient's address
☐ Patient's occupation
☐ Patient's presenting complaint
☐ Compliance with medications
☐ Patient's blood pressures
☐ Presence of weight loss/gain
☐ Amount of weight loss/weight gain
☐ Time period of weight loss/weight gain
☐ Revision of patient's diet
☐ Presence of headaches
☐ Presence of dizziness
☐ Presence of changes in vision
☐ Presence of chest pain
☐ Risk factors

□ Family history
□ Hypertension
□ Diabetes
□ Previous heart condition
□ Smoking
□ Alcohol
□ Exercise
□ Occupation
□ Stress at present
□ Medical history
□ Hospital admissions
□ Surgical history
□ Medications

Differential Diagnosis

1. _____   6. _____
2. _____   7. _____
3. _____   8. _____
4. _____   9. _____
5. _____

Physical Examination Checklist

□ Overall assessment
□ Vitals
  □ Temperature
  □ Pulse
  □ Blood pressure—assess for hypertension
  □ Respirations
□ Examine the neck
  □ Examine JVP wave pattern
  □ Measure the JVP
  □ Assess hepatojugular reflux
  □ Carotid arteries—assess for bruits
□ Cardiovascular system

- ☐ Inspect the precordium
  - ☐ Shape
  - ☐ Scars
  - ☐ Pulses
  - ☐ Apex
- ☐ Palpate the precordium
  - ☐ Tenderness
  - ☐ Pulses
  - ☐ Apex
  - ☐ Thrills
  - ☐ Heaves
- ☐ Percuss the heart borders
- ☐ Auscultate with the bell
  - ☐ Aortic area
  - ☐ Pulmonic area
  - ☐ Erb's point
  - ☐ Tricuspid area
  - ☐ Apex (mitral) area
- ☐ Auscultate with the diaphragm
  - ☐ Aortic area
  - ☐ Pulmonic area
  - ☐ Erb's point
  - ☐ Tricuspid area
  - ☐ Apex (mitral) area
- ☐ Auscultate with the bell—patient in left lateral recumbent position
- ☐ Auscultate with the diaphragm—patient in aortic position
- ☐ Examine the eyes
  - ☐ Alignment
  - ☐ Lid swelling
  - ☐ Lid lesions
  - ☐ Lid retraction
  - ☐ Check visual acuity
  - ☐ Check peripheral visual fields
  - ☐ Examine anterior chamber
  - ☐ Examine the iris
  - ☐ Examine the pupils
- ☐ Opthalmoscopic examination
  - ☐ Retinal hemorrhages
  - ☐ Microaneurysms

☐ Neovascularization
☐ Hard exudates
☐ A full abdominal examination should be performed, if time permits

Physical Examination Findings

General: 45-year-old male, no acute distress
Vitals:

Pulse—82/minute   Temperature—98.8°F
BP—154/92 mm Hg   Respirations—12/minute

Neck:

No JVP noted
No hepatojugular reflux noted
No carotid bruits appreciated

Cardiovascular system:

Precordium normal shape, and size
No abnormal pulsations appreciated
Apical, suprasternal, and abdominal pulsations observed
No tenderness to palpation
Apical, suprasternal, and abdominal pulsations all palpable
No thrills or heaves
S1, S2 heard, no murmurs

Eyes:

No asymmetry noted
No lid swellings, lesions, or retractions noted
Visual acuity 20/40 in left eye, 20/20 in right eye, 20/20 in both eyes
Anterior chamber clear
Pupils equal and reactive to light and accommodation bilaterally
No lens opacities noted
No retinal hemorrhages, microaneurysms, neovascularization, or hard
    exudates noted

Differential Diagnosis

1. _____   3. _____
2. _____   4. _____

Follow-Up

1. _____   4. _____
2. _____   5. _____
3. _____

See Section III for differential diagnosis, appropriate follow-up, and brief case review.

A 19-year-old female complains of severe pain in her abdomen which started 1 day ago. She has also been experiencing some pelvic discomfort.

She describes the pain as a burning pain which moves along her right side to her back. She states that she has been having some difficulty urinating. She finds that she is going to the bathroom frequently, but is only able to pass small amounts of urine. She has noticed that when she does pass urine she feels a burning sensation. The color of her urine is darker that normal, has a foul odor, and at times has some dark red blood in it. She has never experienced these symptoms before. She denies nausea, vomiting, and fever. She has been very healthy in the past. She denies vaginal discharge although does admit that she is sexually active with multiple partners. She has had no pregnancies. Her family history is unremarkable. She smokes approximately half a pack of cigarettes per day and denies the use of alcohol.

Patient History Checklist

- ☐ Patient's name
- ☐ Patient's age
- ☐ Patient's address
- ☐ Patient's occupation
- ☐ Patient's presenting complaint.
- ☐ Absence/presence of abdominal pain
- ☐ History of the pain
    - ☐ Site
    - ☐ Onset
    - ☐ Duration
    - ☐ Intensity
    - ☐ Radiation
    - ☐ Character
    - ☐ Exacerbating factors
    - ☐ Relieving factors

- ☐ Changes in bowel movements
- ☐ Changes in appetite (increased/decreased)
- ☐ Changes in menstrual cycle
- ☐ Frequency of micturition
- ☐ Presence of dysuria
- ☐ Presence of nocturia
- ☐ Presence of hematuria
- ☐ Previous episodes of similar symptoms
- ☐ Presence of vaginal discharge
- ☐ Sexual history
  - ☐ Age of menarche
  - ☐ Frequency of periods
  - ☐ Last menstrual period
  - ☐ Duration of periods
  - ☐ Presence of dysmenorrhea
  - ☐ Presence of dyspareunia
  - ☐ Age of menopause (if relevant)
  - ☐ Sexual activity
  - ☐ History of sexually transmitted diseases
  - ☐ Number of sexual partners (past and present)
  - ☐ Practice of safe sex
  - ☐ Number of pregnancies/outcomes of pregnancies
- ☐ Medical history
- ☐ Hospital admissions
- ☐ Surgical history
- ☐ Medications
- ☐ Family history
  - ☐ Kidney disease
  - ☐ Heart disease
  - ☐ Diabetes
  - ☐ Thyroid disease
  - ☐ Cancer
  - ☐ Others
- ☐ Social history
  - ☐ Smoking
  - ☐ Alcohol
  - ☐ Other drug use

Differential Diagnosis

1. _____   6. _____
2. _____   7. _____
3. _____   8. _____
4. _____   9. _____
5. _____

Physical Examination Checklist

☐ Overall assessment
☐ Vitals
    ☐ Temperature—assess for fever
    ☐ Pulse—assess for tachycardia
    ☐ Blood pressure
    ☐ Respirations
☐ Examine the abdomen
    ☐ Inspect
    ☐ Auscultate
    ☐ Light palpation
    ☐ Deep palpation
    ☐ Assess for organomegaly (palpation and percussion)
    ☐ Assess for CVA tenderness
    ☐ Assess for muscular rigidity
    ☐ Assess for referred rebound tenderness
    ☐ Assess for rebound tenderness
    ☐ Rovsing's sign
    ☐ Psoas sign
    ☐ Obturator sign
    ☐ Cutaneous hyperesthesia
☐ Indicate to the patient that you would like to perform a pelvic examination, including vaginal cultures, but will not do so during this examination

Physical Examination Findings

General: 19-year-old female, no acute distress

Vitals:

Pulse — 76/minute   Temperature — 97.3°F

BP — 116/86 mm Hg   Respirations — 12/minute

Abdomen:

No ecchymosis visible

No visible masses

No striae noted

No visible peristalsis

Bowel sounds present in all quadrants

No bruits heard

No friction rubs over the spleen or liver

Mild tenderness to palpation in pelvic region

No hepatosplenomegaly

No CVA tenderness

No referred rebound tenderness noted

No rebound tenderness

Rovsing's sign negative

Psoas sign negative

Obturator sign negative

No cutaneous hyperesthesia

Differential Diagnosis

1. _____   3. _____
2. _____   4. _____

Follow-Up

1. _____   4. _____

2. _____   5. _____

3. _____

See Section III for differential diagnosis, appropriate follow-up, and brief case review.

CASE 31

A 23-year-old female presents with complaints of weight loss and diarrhea.

The patient first noticed these symptoms approximately 4–5 months ago. She has also noticed some changes in her menstrual cycles. She states that she has been experiencing some feelings of anxiety accompanied by palpitations. She also states that she has been feeling very warm despite the cold weather outside. She has no significant medical history. Her appetite has been good and she reports that she is sleeping well. She does not smoke cigarettes and denies the use of alcohol. Her family history is only significant for thyroid disease.

Patient History Checklist

- ☐ Patient's name
- ☐ Patient's age
- ☐ Patient's address
- ☐ Patient's occupation
- ☐ Patient's presenting complaint
- ☐ Character of the stool
- ☐ Frequency of bowel movements
- ☐ Absence/presence of blood/mucus in the stool
- ☐ Absence/presence of abdominal pain
- ☐ Changes in appetite (increased/decreased)
- ☐ History of weight loss
- ☐ Amount of weight loss
- ☐ Time period of weight loss
- ☐ Fatigue
- ☐ Sweating
- ☐ Heat intolerance
- ☐ Palpitations
- ☐ Anxiety

☐ Changes in menstrual cycle
☐ Changes in the eyes
☐ Swellings in the neck
☐ History of rash on the lower extremities
☐ History of vomiting
☐ Medical history
☐ Hospital admissions
☐ Surgical history
☐ Medications
☐ Family history
    ☐ Thyroid disease
    ☐ Heart disease
    ☐ Diabetes
    ☐ Cancer
    ☐ Others
☐ Social history
    ☐ Smoking
    ☐ Alcohol
    ☐ Other drug use

Differential Diagnosis

1. _____   6. _____
2. _____   7. _____
3. _____   8. _____
4. _____   9. _____
5. _____

Physical Examination Checklist

☐ Overall assessment
☐ Vitals
    ☐ Temperature—assess for fever
    ☐ Pulse
        ☐ assess for tachycardia
        ☐ assess for rapid bounding pulses

□ Blood pressure—assess for increased systolic and decreased diastolic pressures (widened pulse pressure)
□ Respirations
□ Examine the eyes
  □ Assess for lid retraction
  □ Assess for lid lag
  □ Assess for exopthalmos
  □ Check pupillary size
  □ Assess for extraocular muscle weakness
□ Examine the neck
  □ Assess for any swellings
  □ Assess for normal thyroid gland
□ Cardiovascular system
  □ Assess for atrial fibrillation
  □ Assess for tachycardia
  □ Assess for an accentuated S1
  □ Assess for systolic ejection murmur
□ Examine the extremities
  □ Assess for excess diaphoresis of the hands
  □ Assess for proximal muscle weakness
  □ Assess for tremor
  □ Assess for brisk tendon reflexes
  □ Assess for pretibial myxedema (swelling and discoloration of the skin on the anterior lower extremities)

Physical Examination Findings

General: 23-year-old female, no acute distress
Vitals:

Pulse—98/minute   Temperature—99.4°F
BP—144/64 mm Hg   Respirations—14/minute

Eyes

No asymmetry noted
No lid swellings, lesions, or retractions noted
No lid lag noted

No exopthalmos noted

Pupils equal and reactive to light and accommodation bilaterally

Extraocular muscles intact

Neck:

No swellings noted

No goiter appreciated

No thyroid nodules appreciated

Cardiovascular system:

Precordium normal shape and size

No abnormal pulsations appreciated

Apical, suprasternal, and abdominal pulsations observed

No tenderness to palpation

Apical, suprasternal, and abdominal pulsations all palpable

No thrills or heaves

S1, S2 heard, no murmurs

Extremites:

No diaphoresis noted

Normal muscle tone noted in all extremities

Normal power observed in all extremities

No tremor noted

Deep tendon reflexes within normal limits

No pretibial myxedema appreciated

Differential Diagnosis

1. _____   3. _____

2. _____   4. _____

Follow-Up

1. _____   4. _____

2. _____   5. _____

3. _____

See Section III for differential diagnosis, appropriate follow-up, and brief case review.

CASE 32

A 14-year-old female presents complaining of abdominal pain.

The patient reports that the pain started 1 day ago at the umbilical area but has since localized to the right lower quadrant. She has vomited 3 times since the onset of the pain and reports that she has had a fever (maximum temperature 101.8°F). She denies any past or current sexual activity and reports that her periods are normal and she has not experienced any vaginal discharge. She has been healthy in the past and never has been admitted to the hospital. She denies any ill contacts and has not traveled recently. There is no significant family history.

Patient History Checklist

- ☐ Patient's name
- ☐ Patient's age
- ☐ Patient's address
- ☐ Patient's occupation
- ☐ Patient's presenting complaint.
- ☐ Absence/presence of abdominal pain
- ☐ History of the pain
    - ☐ Site
    - ☐ Onset
    - ☐ Duration
    - ☐ Intensity
    - ☐ Radiation
    - ☐ Character
    - ☐ Exacerbating factors
    - ☐ Relieving factors
- ☐ Changes in bowel movements
- ☐ Changes in appetite (increased/decreased)
- ☐ Changes in menstrual cycle
- ☐ Frequency of micturition

☐ Presence of dysuria
☐ Presence of nocturia
☐ Presence of hematuria
☐ Medical history
☐ Hospital admissions
☐ Surgical history
☐ Medications
☐ Family history
  ☐ Heart disease
  ☐ Diabetes
  ☐ Thyroid disease
  ☐ Cancer
  ☐ Others
☐ Social history
  ☐ Smoking
  ☐ Alcohol
  ☐ Other drug use
☐ Sexual history
  ☐ Age of menarche
  ☐ Frequency of periods
  ☐ Last menstrual period
  ☐ Duration of periods
  ☐ Presence of dysmenorrhea
  ☐ Presence of dyspareunia
  ☐ Age of menopause (if relevant)
  ☐ Sexual activity
  ☐ History of sexually transmitted diseases
  ☐ Practice of safe sex
  ☐ Number of pregnancies/outcomes of pregnancies

Differential Diagnosis

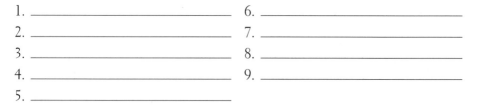

1. _____   6. _____
2. _____   7. _____
3. _____   8. _____
4. _____   9. _____
5. _____

Physical Examination Checklist

☐ Overall assessment
☐ Vitals
    ☐ Temperature—assess for fever
    ☐ Pulse—assess for tachycardia or bradycardia
    ☐ Blood pressure—assess for hypotension
    ☐ Respirations
☐ Examine the eyes
    ☐ Assess for conjunctival pallor
☐ Examine the mouth
    ☐ Assess for signs of dehydration
☐ Examine the abdomen
    ☐ Inspect
    ☐ Auscultate
    ☐ Light palpation
    ☐ Deep palpation
    ☐ Assess for organomegaly (palpation and percussion)
    ☐ Assess for CVA tenderness
    ☐ Assess for muscular rigidity
    ☐ Assess for referred rebound tenderness
    ☐ Assess for rebound tenderness
    ☐ Rovsing's sign
    ☐ Psoas sign
    ☐ Obturator sign
    ☐ Cutaneous hyperesthesia
☐ Indicate to the patient that you would like to perform a digital rectal examination, but will not do so during this examination

Physical Examination Findings

General: 14-year-old female in mild distress
Vitals:

    Pulse—102/minute   Temperature—101.1°F
    BP—108/76 mm Hg   Respirations—16/minute

HEENT:

    Eyes—No conjunctival pallor noted

    Mouth—No crackes/fissures noted; Mucous membranes moist

Abdomen:

    No ecchymosis visible

    No visible masses

    No striae noted

    No visible peristalsis

    Bowel sounds present in all quadrants

    No bruits heard

    No friction rubs over the spleen or liver

    Marked tenderness to palpation in the right lower quadrant

    No hepatosplenomegaly

    No CVA tenderness

    Referred rebound tenderness noted

    Rebound tenderness noted

    Rovsing's sign positive

    Psoas sign positive

    Obturator sign positive

    No cutaneous hyperesthesia noted

Differential Diagnosis

1. _____   3. _____

2. _____   4. _____

Follow-Up

1. _____   4. _____

2. _____   5. _____

3. _____

See Section III for differential diagnosis, appropriate follow-up, and brief case review.

CASE 33

A 29-year-old male is seen in the clinic. He is requesting advice on quitting smoking.

The patient has smoked since the age of 15 and smokes 40 cigarettes per day. He has had repeated attempts at quitting with the longest period of abstinence being 3 weeks. He lives at home with his wife, who also smokes. He finds that the fact that his wife also smokes makes it very difficult for him to quit. In the past he has tried nicotine gum and nicotine patches on different occasions. He has never had any medical problems in the past and has never been hospitalized. He does not use alcohol or any illicit drugs.

Patient History Checklist

- ☐ Patient's name
- ☐ Patient's age
- ☐ Patient's address
- ☐ Patient's occupation
- ☐ Patient's presenting complaint
- ☐ Years of cigarette use
- ☐ Number of cigarettes smoked per day
- ☐ Prior attempts at smoking cessation
- ☐ Prior medications/methods used in past for smoking cessation
- ☐ Partner/friends smoking
- ☐ Presence of productive cough
- ☐ Medical history
- ☐ Hospital admissions
- ☐ Surgical history
- ☐ Medications
- ☐ Family history
  - ☐ Cancer
  - ☐ Heart disease

    ☐ Diabetes
    ☐ Thyroid disease
    ☐ Asthma/allergies
    ☐ Others
☐ Social history
    ☐ Alcohol
    ☐ Other drug use

Differential Diagnosis

1. _____
2. _____
3. _____
4. _____
5. _____

6. _____
7. _____
8. _____
9. _____

Physical Examination Checklist

If a physical examination is required, perform an assessment of the respiratory system

Follow-Up

1. _____
2. _____
3. _____

4. _____
5. _____

See Section III for differential diagnosis, appropriate follow-up, and brief case review.

CASE 34

A 66-year-old male is seen in the outpatient clinic. He has noticed some blood in his stool for the past 3 days.

The patient states that every time he has had a bowel movement for the past 3 days he has seen bright red blood. He does not have any abdominal pain. His appetite is good and has not changed over the 3 days since he has started to see the blood. He has not had any weight loss. He has never noticed anything like this in the past. He states that the blood is mainly on the toilet paper when he wipes following a bowel movement and there is also a small amount on the side of the toilet bowl and in the water. He has not experienced any diarrhea or constipation. He has two bowel movements a day and this is normal for him. He has not had any nausea or vomiting. His medical history is unremarkable. There is a family history of intestinal polyps. There is also a family history of celiac disease and the patient is concerned that he has possibly developed one of these conditions.

Patient History Checklist

- ☐ Patient's name
- ☐ Patient's age
- ☐ Patient's address
- ☐ Patient's occupation
- ☐ Patient's presenting complaint
- ☐ Presence of hematochezia
- ☐ Presence of blood in/on stool
- ☐ Presence of blood on toilet paper
- ☐ Presence of blood in toilet
- ☐ Presence of melena
- ☐ Presence of hematemesis
- ☐ Absence/presence of abdominal pain
- ☐ Presence of weight loss/gain

☐ Amount of weight loss/weight gain
☐ Time period of weight loss/weight gain
☐ Changes in bowel movements
☐ Changes in appetite (increased/decreased)
☐ Presence of rectal pain
☐ Presence of rectal itching/burning
☐ Previous episodes of symptoms
☐ Medical history
☐ Hospital admissions
☐ Surgical history
☐ Medications
☐ Family history
    ☐ Colon cancer
    ☐ Polyps
    ☐ Gastric ulcers
    ☐ Heart disease
    ☐ Diabetes
    ☐ Thyroid disease
    ☐ Cancer
    ☐ Others
☐ Social history
    ☐ Smoking
    ☐ Alcohol
    ☐ Other drug use

Differential Diagnosis

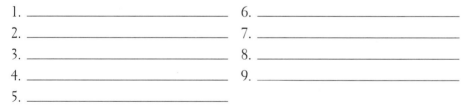

1. _____   6. _____
2. _____   7. _____
3. _____   8. _____
4. _____   9. _____
5. _____

Physical Examination Checklist

- ☐ Overall assessment
- ☐ Vitals
    - ☐ Temperature
    - ☐ Pulse—assess for tachycardia
    - ☐ Blood pressure—assess for hypotension
    - ☐ Respirations
- ☐ Examine the abdomen
    - ☐ Inspect
    - ☐ Auscultate
    - ☐ Light palpation
    - ☐ Deep palpation
    - ☐ Assess for organomegaly (palpation and percussion)
    - ☐ Assess for muscular rigidity
    - ☐ Assess for rebound tenderness
- ☐ Perform a full cardiovascular examination if time permits
- ☐ Indicate to the patient that you would like to perform a digital rectal examination, but will not do so during this examination

Physical Examination Findings

General: 66-year-old male, no acute distress

Vitals:

Pulse—92/minute   Temperature—98.2°F

BP—134/90 mm Hg   Respirations—16/minute

Abdomen:

No ecchymosis visible

No visible masses

No striae noted

No visible peristalsis

Bowel sounds present in all quadrants

No bruits heard

No friction rubs over the spleen or liver

No tenderness to palpation
No hepatosplenomegaly
No rebound tenderness noted

Differential Diagnosis

1. _____   3. _____
2. _____   4. _____

Follow-Up

1. _____   4. _____
2. _____   5. _____
3. _____

See Section III for differential diagnosis, appropriate follow-up, and brief case review.

CASE 35

A 69-year-old male is seen in the emergency department complaining of chest pain.

The pain is located on the left side of his chest and he describes it as a sharp pain, which lasts 30–40 minutes and then subsides. He has been awakened three times in the past week because of the pain. He reports that he first experienced the pain approximately 6 months ago. However, at that time he was experiencing the pain only once in a while and usually while doing his gardening. His medical history is only significant for hypertension, which was first diagnosed 25 years ago. He smokes half a pack of cigarettes per day and has done so for the past 45 years. Both his father and two of his brothers died from heart disease. There is no other significant family history.

Patient History Checklist

- ☐ Patient's name
- ☐ Patient's age
- ☐ Patient's address
- ☐ Patient's occupation
- ☐ Patient's presenting complaint
- ☐ History of the pain
  - ☐ Site
  - ☐ Onset
  - ☐ Duration
  - ☐ Intensity
  - ☐ Radiation
  - ☐ Character
  - ☐ Past experience of this pain
  - ☐ Exacerbating factors
  - ☐ Relieving factors
  - ☐ Medications taken to relieve the pain

☐ Associated factors (sweating, palpitations, shortness of breath, feelings of anxiety, feeling of impending doom)
☐ Pain in relation to meals
☐ Presence of weight loss/gain
☐ Amount of weight loss/weight gain
☐ Time period of weight loss/weight gain
☐ Risk factors
☐ Family history
    ☐ Hypertension
    ☐ Diabetes
    ☐ Previous heart condition
    ☐ Smoking
    ☐ Alcohol
    ☐ Exercise
    ☐ Occupation
    ☐ Stress at present
☐ Medical history
☐ Hospital admissions
☐ Surgical history
☐ Medications

Differential Diagnosis

1. _____   6. _____
2. _____   7. _____
3. _____   8. _____
4. _____   9. _____
5. _____

Physical Examination Checklist

☐ Overall assessment
☐ Vitals
    ☐ Temperature
    ☐ Pulse—assess for tachycardia

- ☐ Blood pressure—assess for hypertension
- ☐ Respirations
☐ Examine the neck
  - ☐ Examine JVP wave pattern
  - ☐ Measure the JVP
  - ☐ Assess hepatojugular reflux
  - ☐ Carotid arteries—assess for bruits
☐ Cardiovascular system
  - ☐ Inspect the precordium
    - ☐ Shape
    - ☐ Scars
    - ☐ Pulses
    - ☐ Apex
  - ☐ Palpate the precordium
    - ☐ Tenderness
    - ☐ Pulses
    - ☐ Apex
    - ☐ Thrills
    - ☐ Heaves
  - ☐ Percuss the heart borders
  - ☐ Auscultate with the bell
    - ☐ Aortic area
    - ☐ Pulmonic area
    - ☐ Erb's point
    - ☐ Tricuspid area
    - ☐ Apex (mitral) area
  - ☐ Auscultate with the diaphragm
    - ☐ Aortic area
    - ☐ Pulmonic area
    - ☐ Erb's point
    - ☐ Tricuspid area
    - ☐ Apex (mitral) area
  - ☐ Auscultate with the bell—patient in left lateral recumbent position
  - ☐ Auscultate with the diaphragm—patient in aortic position
☐ A full examination of the respiratory system should be performed, if time permits

Physical Examination Findings

General: 69-year-old male, no acute distress
Vitals:

Pulse—68/minute Temperature—98.2°F
BP—154/92 mm Hg Respirations—16/minute

Neck:

No JVP noted
No hepatojugular reflux noted
No carotid bruits appreciated

Cardiovascular system:

Precordium normal shape, and size
No abnormal pulsations appreciated
Apical, suprasternal, and abdominal pulsations observed
No tenderness to palpation
Apical, suprasternal, and abdominal pulsations all palpable
No thrills or heaves
S1, S2 heard, no murmurs

Differential Diagnosis

1. _____ 3. _____
2. _____ 4. _____

Follow-Up

1. _____ 4. _____
2. _____ 5. _____
3. _____

See Section III for differential diagnosis, appropriate follow-up, and brief case review.

CASE 36

A 29-year-old male is seen in the outpatient clinic. He has been feeling tired and generally unwell for the past 6 months.

The patient is vague about his symptoms and obtaining a history proves to be a difficult task. On further questioning, the patient becomes very agitated and defensive. He is currently unemployed and lives alone. When questioned about drug and alcohol use the patient becomes further agitated and demands that something be done to make him feel better. When questioned still further, the patient admits that he has been using cocaine for the past year and has been drinking daily for the past 3 years. He states that he is ready for a change in his lifestyle, but requires help in doing so. He currently drinks approximately one bottle of vodka per day and smokes 2 packs of cigarettes per day. He is unsure exactly how much cocaine he uses per day but states that it is a lot.

Patient History Checklist

- ☐ Patient's name
- ☐ Patient's age
- ☐ Patient's address
- ☐ Patient's occupation
- ☐ Patient's presenting complaint
- ☐ Duration of symptoms
- ☐ Social history
  - ☐ Smoking (how much?)
  - ☐ Alcohol (how much?) (CAGE questions)
  - ☐ Drug use (Specific drugs, including method of use)
  - ☐ Family situation
  - ☐ Work situation
  - ☐ Ability to function at work
  - ☐ Ability to function at home
  - ☐ Presence of support system

- ☐ Presence of fatigue
- ☐ Presence of irritability
- ☐ Difficulty concentrating
- ☐ Difficulty sleeping
- ☐ Presence of palpitations
- ☐ Loss of appetite
- ☐ Presence of weight loss/gain
- ☐ Amount of weight loss/weight gain
- ☐ Time period of weight loss/weight gain
- ☐ Medical history
- ☐ Hospital admissions
- ☐ Surgical history
- ☐ Medications
- ☐ Sexual history
  - ☐ Number of sexual partners
  - ☐ History of sexually transmitted diseases
  - ☐ Use of condoms
  - ☐ HIV status
- ☐ Suicidal ideation
  - ☐ Suicide plan
  - ☐ Previous suicide attempts
- ☐ Family history
  - ☐ Drug abuse
  - ☐ Depression
  - ☐ Psychiatric illnesses
  - ☐ Heart disease
  - ☐ Diabetes
  - ☐ Thyroid disease
  - ☐ Cancer
  - ☐ Others

Differential Diagnosis

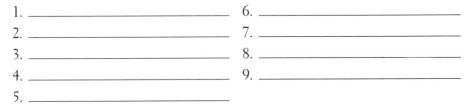

1. _____   6. _____
2. _____   7. _____
3. _____   8. _____
4. _____   9. _____
5. _____

Physical Examination Checklist

☐ Overall assessment
☐ Vitals
   ☐ Temperature
   ☐ Pulse—assess for tachycardia
   ☐ Blood pressure—assess for hypertension
   ☐ Respirations
☐ Examine the mouth—assess for signs of nutritional deficiencies
☐ Examine the eyes—assess for conjunctival pallor
☐ Examine the neck
   ☐ Examine JVP wave pattern
   ☐ Measure the JVP
   ☐ Assess hepatojugular reflux
   ☐ Carotid arteries—assess for bruits
☐ Cardiovascular system
   ☐ Inspect the precordium
      ☐ Shape
      ☐ Scars
      ☐ Pulses
      ☐ Apex
   ☐ Palpate the precordium
      ☐ Tenderness
      ☐ Pulses
      ☐ Apex
      ☐ Thrill
      ☐ Heaves
   ☐ Percuss the heart borders
   ☐ Auscultate with the bell
      ☐ Aortic area
      ☐ Pulmonic area
      ☐ Erb's point
      ☐ Tricuspid area
      ☐ Apex (mitral) area
   ☐ Auscultate with the diaphragm
      ☐ Aortic area
      ☐ Pulmonic area
      ☐ Erb's point

☐ Tricuspid area
☐ Apex (mitral) area
☐ Auscultate with the bell—patient in left lateral recumbent position
☐ Auscultate with the diaphragm—patient in aortic position
☐ Examine the abdomen
    ☐ Inspect
    ☐ Auscultate
    ☐ Light palpation
    ☐ Deep palpation
    ☐ Assess for organomegaly (palpation and percussion)
    ☐ Assess for muscular rigidity
    ☐ Assess for rebound tenderness
    ☐ Assess for signs of liver failure (hepatomegaly, spider angiomas, gyneco-mastia, caput medusa, ascites)
☐ If time permits, perform an examination of the central nervous system, paying particular attention to the pupils
☐ Perform a complete physical examination, if time permits, to assess for other features of drug/alcohol abuse

Physical Examination Findings

General: 29-year-old male, agitated appearing
Vitals:

    Pulse—102/minute   Temperature—99.1°F
    BP—152/96 mm Hg   Respirations—18/minute

Eyes—No conjunctival pallor noted
Mouth—No cracks/fissures noted; no pallor
Neck:

    No JVP noted
    No hepatojugular reflux noted
    No carotid bruits appreciated

Cardiovascular system:

    Precordium normal shape, and size
    No abnormal pulsations appreciated
    Apical, suprasternal, and abdominal pulsations observed

No tenderness to palpation

Apical, suprasternal, and abdominal pulsations all palpable

No thrills or heaves

S1, S2 heard, no murmurs

Abdomen:

No ecchymosis visible

No visible masses

No striae noted

No visible peristalsis

No spider angiomas

No gynecomastia

No caput medusa

Bowel sounds present in all quadrants

No bruits heard

No friction rubs over the spleen or liver

No tenderness to palpation

No hepatosplenomegaly

No rebound tenderness

No shifting dullness

No fluid wave

Differential Diagnosis

1. _____   3. _____
2. _____   4. _____

Follow-Up

1. _____   4. _____
2. _____   5. _____
3. _____

See Section III for differential diagnosis, appropriate follow-up, and brief case review.

CASE 37

A 14-year-old male is brought to the emergency department by his mother. He is complaining of severe chest pain.

The chest pain is bilateral and does not seem to be associated with breathing or with movement. He was diagnosed with sickle-cell anemia at the age of 4. He has approximately one painful crisis per year usually brought on by physical exercise. The patient reports that he had been running and playing in the school yard prior to this episode. He also complains that he is experiencing some bilateral leg pain. He is feeling fatigued and slightly short of breath.

Patient History Checklist

- ☐ Patient's name
- ☐ Patient's age
- ☐ Patient's address
- ☐ Patient's occupation
- ☐ Patient's presenting complaint
- ☐ Absence/presence of pain
- ☐ History of the pain
  - ☐ Site
  - ☐ Onset
  - ☐ Duration
  - ☐ Intensity
  - ☐ Radiation
  - ☐ Character
  - ☐ Exacerbating factors
  - ☐ Relieving factors
  - ☐ Medications used to relieve symptoms
- ☐ Presence of pain on movement
- ☐ Swelling of the affected area
- ☐ Previous episodes of symptoms

- ☐ Presence of fatigue
- ☐ Presence of shortness of breath
- ☐ Presence of nausea/vomiting
- ☐ Presence of fever
- ☐ Presence of hematuria
- ☐ Presence of frequent urination
- ☐ Presence of excessive thirst
- ☐ History of trauma
- ☐ History of recent surgery
- ☐ History of unusual exercise
- ☐ Presence of sickle-cell disease complications
- ☐ Presence of cough
- ☐ Medical history
- ☐ Hospital admissions
- ☐ Surgical history
- ☐ Medications
- ☐ Family history
  - ☐ Sickle-cell disease
  - ☐ Sickle-cell trait
  - ☐ Rheumatoid arthritis
  - ☐ Heart disease
  - ☐ Diabetes
  - ☐ Thyroid disease
  - ☐ Cancer
  - ☐ Others
- ☐ Social history
  - ☐ Smoking
  - ☐ Alcohol
  - ☐ Other drug use

Differential Diagnosis

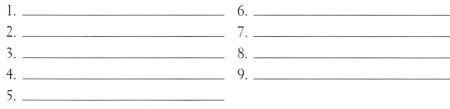

1. _____   6. _____
2. _____   7. _____
3. _____   8. _____
4. _____   9. _____
5. _____

Physical Examination Checklist

- ☐ Overall assessment
- ☐ Vitals
  - ☐ Temperature—assess for fever
  - ☐ Pulse—assess for tachycardia
  - ☐ Blood pressure
  - ☐ Respirations—assess for tachypnea
- ☐ Observe patient's gait
- ☐ Cardiovascular system
  - ☐ Inspect the precordium
    - ☐ Shape
    - ☐ Scars
    - ☐ Pulses
    - ☐ Apex
  - ☐ Palpate the precordium
    - ☐ Tenderness
    - ☐ Pulses
    - ☐ Apex
    - ☐ Thrills
    - ☐ Heaves
  - ☐ Percuss the heart borders
  - ☐ Auscultate with the bell
    - ☐ Aortic area
    - ☐ Pulmonic area
    - ☐ Erb's point
    - ☐ Tricuspid area
    - ☐ Apex (mitral) area
  - ☐ Auscultate with the diaphragm
    - ☐ Aortic area
    - ☐ Pulmonic area
    - ☐ Erb's point
    - ☐ Tricuspid area
    - ☐ Apex (mitral) area
  - ☐ Auscultate with the bell—patient in left lateral recumbent position
  - ☐ Auscultate with the diaphragm—patient in aortic position
- ☐ Examine the extremities (bilaterally)
  - ☐ Inspect upper extremities

- ☐ Symmetry
- ☐ Deformities
- ☐ Swellings
- ☐ Areas of erythema
- ☐ Palpate upper extremities
  - ☐ Temperature
  - ☐ Tenderness
  - ☐ Masses
- ☐ Inspect lower extremities
  - ☐ Symmetry
  - ☐ Deformities
  - ☐ Swellings
  - ☐ Ulcers
  - ☐ Areas of erythema
- ☐ Palpate lower extremities
  - ☐ Temperature
  - ☐ Tenderness
  - ☐ Masses

Physical Examination Findings

General: 14-year-old male, uncomfortable appearing

Vitals:

Pulse—108/minute   Temperature—97.3°F

BP—132/84 mm Hg   Respirations—18/minute

No abnormal gait observed

Cardiovascular system:

Precordium normal shape, and size

No abnormal pulsations appreciated

Apical, suprasternal, and abdominal pulsations observed

No tenderness to palpation

Apical, suprasternal, and abdominal pulsations all palpable

No thrills or heaves

S1, S2 heard, no murmurs

Upper extremities:

    Symmetrical

    No ecchymosis, erythema, swellings, or deformities noted

    No tenderness on palpation

    Temperature equal bilaterally

Lower extremities:

    Symmetrical

    No ecchymosis, erythema, swellings, or deformities noted

    No ulcers noted

    No tenderness on palpation

    Temperature equal bilaterally

Differential Diagnosis

1. _____   3. _____

2. _____   4. _____

Follow-Up

1. _____   4. _____

2. _____   5. _____

3. _____

See Section III for differential diagnosis, appropriate follow-up, and brief case review.

CASE 38

A 65-year-old male is seen in the clinic. He has been having intermittent chest pain over the past 4–6 months.

The pain is located on the left side of his chest and occasionally radiates to his left arm. He describes the pain as a squeezing sensation, which lasts approximately 25–30 minutes and then subsides. He mainly gets the pain while doing his garden work and denies ever having experienced the pain while at rest. He denies any associated symptoms including shortness of breath, diaphoresis, nausea, or vomiting. He has a medical history significant for hypertension and hypercholesterolemia.

Patient History Checklist

- ☐ Patient's name
- ☐ Patient's age
- ☐ Patient's address
- ☐ Patient's occupation
- ☐ Patient's presenting complaint
- ☐ History of the pain
  - ☐ Site
  - ☐ Onset
  - ☐ Duration
  - ☐ Intensity
  - ☐ Radiation
  - ☐ Character
  - ☐ Past experience of this pain
  - ☐ Exacerbating factors
  - ☐ Relieving factors
  - ☐ Medications taken to relieve the pain
- ☐ Associated factors (sweating, palpitations, shortness of breath, feelings of anxiety, feeling of impending doom)

☐ Pain in relation to meals
☐ Presence of weight loss/gain
☐ Amount of weight loss/weight gain
☐ Time period of weight loss/weight gain
☐ Risk factors
    ☐ Family history
    ☐ Hypertension
    ☐ Diabetes
    ☐ Previous heart condition
    ☐ Smoking
    ☐ Alcohol
    ☐ Exercise
    ☐ Occupation
    ☐ Stress at present
☐ Medical history
☐ Hospital admissions
☐ Surgical history
☐ Medications

Differential Diagnosis

1. _____   6. _____
2. _____   7. _____
3. _____   8. _____
4. _____   9. _____
5. _____

Physical Examination Checklist

☐ Overall assessment
☐ Vitals
    ☐ Temperature
    ☐ Pulse—assess for tachycardia
    ☐ Blood pressure—assess for hypertension
    ☐ Respirations
☐ Examine the neck

- ☐ Examine JVP wave pattern
- ☐ Measure the JVP
- ☐ Assess hepatojugular reflux
- ☐ Carotid arteries—assess for bruits
☐ Cardiovascular system
  - ☐ Inspect the precordium
    - ☐ Shape
    - ☐ Scars
    - ☐ Pulses
    - ☐ Apex
  - ☐ Palpate the precordium
    - ☐ Tenderness
    - ☐ Pulses
    - ☐ Apex
    - ☐ Thrills
    - ☐ Heaves
  - ☐ Percuss the heart borders
  - ☐ Auscultate with the bell
    - ☐ Aortic area
    - ☐ Pulmonic area
    - ☐ Erb's point
    - ☐ Tricuspid area
    - ☐ Apex (mitral) area
  - ☐ Auscultate with the diaphragm
    - ☐ Aortic area
    - ☐ Pulmonic area
    - ☐ Erb's point
    - ☐ Tricuspid area
    - ☐ Apex (mitral) area
  - ☐ Auscultate with the bell—patient in left lateral recumbent position
  - ☐ Auscultate with the diaphragm—patient in aortic position

Physical Examination Findings

General: 64-year-old male, no acute distress
Vitals:

Pulse—68/minute   Temperature—97.4°F
BP—148/96 mm Hg   Respirations—14/minute

Neck:

No JVP noted
No hepatojugular reflux noted
No carotid bruits appreciated

Cardiovascular system:

Precordium normal shape and size
No abnormal pulsations appreciated
Apical, suprasternal, and abdominal pulsations observed
No tenderness to palpation
Apical, suprasternal, and abdominal pulsations all palpable
No thrills or heaves
S1, S2 heard, no murmurs

Differential Diagnosis

1. _____   3. _____
2. _____   4. _____

Follow-Up

1. _____   4. _____
2. _____   5. _____
3. _____

See Section III for differential diagnosis, appropriate follow-up, and brief case review.

CASE 39

A 33-year-old female is seen in the clinic. She has amenorrhea and states that she thinks that she might be pregnant.

The patient's last menstrual period was 5 weeks ago. She states that her periods are very regular and occur every 28 days. She has been married to her husband for 3 years. She has been trying to get pregnant and she really hopes that she is indeed pregnant at this time. She has been having unprotected intercourse with her husband for the past 2 years; however she did not achieved pregnancy thus far. She has been healthy in the past and has never been admitted to the hospital for any reason. She has no children and has never been pregnant.

Patient History Checklist

- ☐ Patient's name
- ☐ Patient's age
- ☐ Patient's address
- ☐ Patient's occupation
- ☐ Patient's presenting complaint
- ☐ Sexual history
    - ☐ Last menstrual period
    - ☐ Age of menarche
    - ☐ Frequency of periods
    - ☐ Duration of periods
    - ☐ History of sexually transmitted diseases
    - ☐ Presence of vaginal discharge
    - ☐ Presence of vaginal bleeding/spotting
    - ☐ Presence of dyspareunia
    - ☐ Number of pregnancies/outcomes of pregnancies
    - ☐ Number of abortions
    - ☐ Reasons for abortions

- ☐ Presence of weight gain
- ☐ Amount of weight gain
- ☐ Time period of weight gain
- ☐ Presence of breast tenderness
- ☐ Presence of breast enlargement
- ☐ Presence of nipple discharge
- ☐ Presence of morning sickness
- ☐ Presence of fatigue
- ☐ Partner's details
  - ☐ Age
  - ☐ Occupation
  - ☐ History of sexually transmitted diseases
  - ☐ Number of children, if any
- ☐ Medical history
- ☐ Hospital admissions
- ☐ Surgical history
- ☐ Medications
- ☐ Family history
  - ☐ Siblings with children
  - ☐ Depression
  - ☐ Psychiatric illnesses
  - ☐ Heart disease
  - ☐ Diabetes
  - ☐ Thyroid disease
  - ☐ Cancer
  - ☐ Others
- ☐ Social history
  - ☐ Smoking
  - ☐ Alcohol
  - ☐ Other drug use
  - ☐ Family situation
  - ☐ Feelings of anxiety
  - ☐ Exercise
  - ☐ Diet

Differential Diagnosis

1. _____   6. _____
2. _____   7. _____
3. _____   8. _____
4. _____   9. _____
5. _____

Physical Examination Checklist

- ☐ Overall assessment
- ☐ Vitals
  - ☐ Temperature
  - ☐ Pulse
  - ☐ Blood pressure
  - ☐ Respirations
- ☐ Examine the abdomen
  - ☐ Inspect
  - ☐ Auscultate
  - ☐ Light palpation
  - ☐ Deep palpation
  - ☐ Assess for organomegaly (palpation and percussion)
  - ☐ Assess for pelvic abdominal masses/fundal height
  - ☐ Assess for fetal movements
- ☐ Indicate to the patient that you would like to perform a breast examination and a pelvic examination, but will not do so during this examination

Physical Examination Findings

General: 33-year-old female, no acute distress
Vitals:

Pulse—68/minute	Temperature—97.8°F
BP—110/68 mm Hg	Respirations—14/minute

Abdomen:

> No ecchymosis visible
> No visible masses
> No striae noted
> No visible peristalsis
> Bowel sounds present in all quadrants
> No bruits heard
> No friction rubs over the spleen or liver
> No tenderness to palpation
> No hepatosplenomegaly
> Fundus not palpable
> No fetal movements appreciated

Differential Diagnosis

1. _____   3. _____
2. _____   4. _____

Follow-Up

1. _____   4. _____
2. _____   5. _____
3. _____

See Section III for differential diagnosis, appropriate follow-up, and brief case review.

CASE 40

A 65-year-old female is seen in the emergency department complaining of a cough for the past 3 days.

The patient was brought to the emergency department by her daughter. She has had a productive cough for the past 3 days. Her sputum is yellow/green. She has also been experiencing some difficulty breathing since the onset of the cough. She has had intermittent chest pain related to the coughing. She has been febrile at home with a temperature ranging from 99–101°F. Her only significant medical history is arthritis, which she developed at a young age. She is fairly disabled from this at this point. She has a difficult time getting around and relies on her daughter to help her with most daily activities including dressing and using the toilet. She has had no ill contacts that she is aware of. She has never experienced these symptoms before.

Patient History Checklist

- ☐ Patient's name
- ☐ Patient's age
- ☐ Patient's address
- ☐ Patient's occupation
- ☐ Patient's presenting complaint
- ☐ Duration of symptoms
- ☐ Presence of cough (productive/nonproductive)
- ☐ Appearance of the sputum
- ☐ Presence of blood in the sputum
- ☐ Shortness of breath
- ☐ Presence of fever
- ☐ Presence of rhinorrhea
- ☐ Presence of chest pain
- ☐ History of the pain

- ☐ Site
- ☐ Onset
- ☐ Duration
- ☐ Intensity
- ☐ Radiation
- ☐ Character
- ☐ Exacerbating factors
- ☐ Relieving factors
- ☐ Nausea/vomiting
- ☐ History of weight loss
- ☐ Amount of weight loss
- ☐ Time period of weight loss
- ☐ Presence of night sweats
- ☐ Ill contacts
- ☐ Medical history
- ☐ Hospital admissions
- ☐ Surgical history
- ☐ Medications
- ☐ Family history
  - ☐ Cancer
  - ☐ Heart disease
  - ☐ Diabetes
  - ☐ Thyroid disease
  - ☐ Asthma/allergies
  - ☐ Others
- ☐ Social history
  - ☐ Smoking
  - ☐ Alcohol
  - ☐ Other drug use

Differential Diagnosis

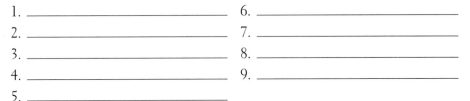

1. _____   6. _____
2. _____   7. _____
3. _____   8. _____
4. _____   9. _____
5. _____

Physical Examination Checklist

- ☐ Overall assessment
- ☐ Vitals
    - ☐ Temperature—assess for fever
    - ☐ Pulse—assess for tachycardia
    - ☐ Blood pressure—assess for hypotension
    - ☐ Respirations—assess for tachypnea
- ☐ Examine the face—assess mucus membranes for the presence of cyanosis
- ☐ Examine the neck
    - ☐ Assess for lymphadenopathy
    - ☐ Assess for use of accessory muscles
    - ☐ Assess the position of the trachea
- ☐ Examine the extremities
    - ☐ Assess for clubbing
    - ☐ Assess for cyanosis
- ☐ Respiratory system—examine the thorax
    - ☐ Inspect
        - ☐ Size
        - ☐ Shape
        - ☐ Symmetry
        - ☐ Movement
        - ☐ Deformities of the ribs
        - ☐ Deformities of the spine
        - ☐ Scars
    - ☐ Palpate
        - ☐ Tenderness
        - ☐ Excursion
        - ☐ Tactile fremitus
        - ☐ Chest dimensions
        - ☐ Position of the diaphragm
    - ☐ Percuss
        - ☐ All areas comparing side to side
        - ☐ Diaphragm excursion (left)
        - ☐ Diaphragm excursion (right)
    - ☐ Auscultate
        - ☐ All areas comparing side to side
        - ☐ Breath sounds

☐ Vocal resonance
☐ Whispering pectoriloquy
☐ Aegophony

Physical Examination Findings

General: 65-year-old female in mild respiratory distress
Vitals:

Pulse — 108/minute	Temperature — 101.8°F
BP — 110/68 mm Hg	Respirations — 28/minute

HEENT: Mouth — Mucous membranes moist; no cyanosis noted
Neck:

No lymphadenopathy

Some use of accessory muscles of respirations

Trachea midline

Extremities: No clubbing or cyanosis noted

Respiratory system:

Thorax normal size and shape

No asymmetry noted

No scars or deformities noted

No tenderness to palpation

Tactile fremitus increased at left base

No increased anteroposterior diameter

Dull to percussion at left base

Level of the diaphragms equal bilaterally

Decreased breath sounds appreciated at left base

No wheezing noted

Whispering pectoriloquy noted at left base

Positive aegophony noted at left base

Differential Diagnosis

1. _____   3. _____
2. _____   4. _____

Follow-Up

1. _____   4. _____
2. _____   5. _____
3. _____

See Section III for differential diagnosis, appropriate follow-up, and brief case review.

CASE 41

A 40-year-old male patient is seen in the clinic complaining of pain in his hands, his feet, and his right leg.

The patient reports that he was recently hospitalized following a collapse at work. He was discharged from the hospital 3 days ago. He is now experiencing pain and loss of sensation in his hands, feet, and right leg. The patient further reports that he has had these symptoms in the past, some years ago, and at that time these were relieved with bed rest and fluids. The patient describes the pain as a burning sensation. He denies fever, his appetite is good, and he has not noticed any weight loss. He has no significant medical history. He denies the use of cigarettes. He reluctantly admits that he drinks approximately one bottle of rum a day and has done so for the past 15 years.

Patient History Checklist

☐ Patient's name
☐ Patient's age
☐ Patient's address
☐ Patient's occupation (details of all current and previous occupations with any toxin or chemical exposure)
☐ Patient's presenting complaint
☐ History of the pain
    ☐ Site
    ☐ Onset
    ☐ Duration
    ☐ Intensity
    ☐ Radiation
    ☐ Character
    ☐ Exacerbating factors
    ☐ Relieving factors

☐ Decreased sensation
☐ Changes in bowel movements
☐ Changes in appetite (increased/decreased)
☐ Weight gain/loss
☐ Amount of weight loss/weight gain
☐ Time period of weight loss/weight gain
☐ Dietary history
☐ Medical history
☐ Hospital admissions
☐ Surgical history
☐ Medications
☐ Family history
   ☐ Heart disease
   ☐ Diabetes
   ☐ Thyroid disease
   ☐ Cancer
   ☐ Others
☐ Social history
   ☐ Smoking
   ☐ Alcohol (CAGE questions)
   ☐ Other drug use

Differential Diagnosis

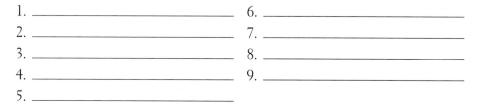

1. _____   6. _____
2. _____   7. _____
3. _____   8. _____
4. _____   9. _____
5. _____

Physical Examination Checklist

☐ Overall assessment
☐ Vitals
   ☐ Temperature
   ☐ Pulse

- ☐ Blood pressure
- ☐ Respirations
☐ Evaluate mental status
  - ☐ Orientation to person, place, and time
  - ☐ Level of consciousness
  - ☐ Short-term memory
  - ☐ Long-term memory
  - ☐ Observe the patient's gait and speech
☐ Examine the head — assess for masses, ecchymosis, lacerations, tenderness
☐ Examine the ears
  - ☐ Assess the external ear canal for fluid drainage
  - ☐ Assess the tympanic membranes
☐ Examine the eyes — assess for conjunctival pallor
☐ Examine the mouth — assess for signs of nutritional deficiencies
☐ Examine all cranial nerves (I–XII)
☐ Examine the sensory system
  - ☐ Check for pain and crude touch in all parts of the body
  - ☐ Romberg's test
  - ☐ Proprioception at fingers and toes
  - ☐ Vibratory sense
  - ☐ Stereognosis
  - ☐ Graphesthesia
  - ☐ 2-point discrimination
  - ☐ Point localization
  - ☐ Extinction
☐ Examine the motor system
  - ☐ Inspect the motor system for atrophy, fasciculations, and involuntary movements
  - ☐ Palpate all limbs for muscle tone
  - ☐ Check all major muscle groups for power
  - ☐ Check all reflexes
    - ☐ Abdominal
    - ☐ Plantar
    - ☐ Biceps
    - ☐ Triceps
    - ☐ Brachioradialis
    - ☐ Knee
    - ☐ Ankle

☐ Examine the cerebellum
  ☐ Ask the patient to walk in a straight line, heel to toe
  ☐ Ask the patient to walk in a straight line on his/her heels
  ☐ Ask the patient to walk in a straight line on his/her toes
  ☐ Ask the patient to perform the finger–nose test
  ☐ Ask the patient to perform the knee–heel–shin test
  ☐ Check for dysdiadochokinesia
☐ If time permits, perform a full abdominal examination to assess for signs of malnutrition and liver disease/failure

Physical Examination Findings

General: 40-year-old male, no acute distress

Vitals:

Pulse — 82/minute	Temperature — 97.9°F
BP — 142/86 mm Hg	Respirations — 14/minute

Mental status:

Patient oriented to person, place, and time

Patient awake and alert

Short- and long-term memory intact

No abnormal gait observed

Speech appropriate

HEENT:

Head — No masses, ecchymosis, lacerations, or tenderness appreciated

Ears — No drainage noted; tympanic membranes visualized bilaterally

Eyes — No conjunctival pallor noted

Mouth — No cracks/fissures noted; no pallor

Cranial nerves: I–XII intact

Sensory system: Sensation intact bilaterally

Motor system:

No atrophy noted

No fasciculations

Normal muscle tone noted in all extremities

Decreased power observed in upper extremities bilaterally (3/5) and right lower extremity (3/5)

Deep tendon reflexes intact

Abdominal reflex present

Plantar reflex down going

Cerebellum: No abnormalities noted

Differential Diagnosis

1. _____   3. _____
2. _____   4. _____

Follow-Up

1. _____   4. _____
2. _____   5. _____
3. _____

See Section III for differential diagnosis, appropriate follow-up, and brief case review.

CASE 42

A 48-year-old female presents to the outpatient clinic complaining of fatigue.

She reports that the fatigue began several months ago. She states that she has also been feeling "a bit depressed" recently and finds that she is having some difficulty concentrating. On further questioning, she tells you that she also has been constipated over the past few months and has gained approximately 16 lbs despite noticing a decrease in her appetite. She has noticed that her hair has become brittle and finds that her skin is very dry. She has no significant medical history. She lives at home with her husband and their two children and is a stay-at-home mom.

Patient History Checklist

- ☐ Patient's name
- ☐ Patient's age
- ☐ Patient's address
- ☐ Patient's occupation
- ☐ Patient's presenting complaint.
- ☐ Duration of symptoms
- ☐ History of weight gain
- ☐ Amount of weight gain
- ☐ Time period of weight gain
- ☐ Fatigue
- ☐ Psychiatric evaluation
    - ☐ Loss of interest in usual activities
    - ☐ Difficulty concentrating
    - ☐ Agitation
    - ☐ Feelings of worthlessness
    - ☐ Delusions/hallucinations
    - ☐ Suicidal ideation

- ☐ Frequency of bowel movements
- ☐ Constipation
- ☐ Swelling around eyes
- ☐ Swelling of the lower extremities
- ☐ Changes in appetite (increased/decreased)
- ☐ Changes in sleep patterns
- ☐ Cold intolerance
- ☐ Difficulty swallowing
- ☐ Changes in menstrual cycle
- ☐ Hair changes
- ☐ Voice changes
- ☐ History of treatment for hyperthyroidism
- ☐ Swellings in neck
- ☐ Medical history, including any psychiatric illness
- ☐ Hospital admissions
- ☐ Surgical history
- ☐ Medications
- ☐ Family history
  - ☐ Thyroid disease
  - ☐ Heart disease
  - ☐ Diabetes
  - ☐ Cancer
  - ☐ Psychiatric disorders
  - ☐ Others
- ☐ Social history
  - ☐ Smoking
  - ☐ Alcohol
  - ☐ Other drug use (especially lithium)

Differential Diagnosis

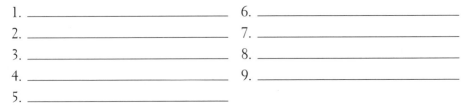

1. _____   6. _____
2. _____   7. _____
3. _____   8. _____
4. _____   9. _____
5. _____

Physical Examination Checklist

☐ Overall assessment
☐ Vitals
  ☐ Temperature—assess for hypothermia
  ☐ Pulse—assess for bradycardia
  ☐ Blood pressure—assess for decreased systolic and increased diastolic pressures (narrowed pulse pressure)
  ☐ Respirations
☐ Examine the face
  ☐ Assess for facial swelling
  ☐ Assess for coarse, dry skin
  ☐ Assess for swelling of the tongue
  ☐ Assess for thinning of the scalp hair and eyebrows (laterally)
☐ Examine the eyes
  ☐ Assess for periorbital puffiness
  ☐ Assess for thickening of the eye lids
☐ Examine the neck
  ☐ Assess for any swellings
  ☐ Assess for normal thyroid gland
☐ Examine the cardiovascular system
  ☐ Assess for diminished heart sounds
  ☐ Assess for bradycardia
☐ Examine the extremities
  ☐ Assess for swelling of the hands
  ☐ Assess for muscle weakness
  ☐ Assess for hypoactive tendon reflexes with a slow relaxation phase

Physical Examination Findings

General: 48-year-old female, no acute distress
Vitals:

Pulse—62/minute	Temperature—97.1°F
BP—112/94 mm Hg	Respirations—14/minute

HEENT:

    Head

        No facial swelling

        No dry skin appreciated

        No swelling of the tongue noted

        No thinning of the eyebrows noted

    Eyes

    No periorbital swelling noted

    No thickening/swelling of the eyelids noted

Neck:

    No swellings noted

    No goiter appreciated

    No thyroid nodules appreciated

Cardiovascular system:

    Precordium normal shape and size

    No abnormal pulsations appreciated

    Apical, suprasternal, and abdominal pulsations observed

    No tenderness to palpation

    Apical, suprasternal, and abdominal pulsations all palpable

    No thrills or heaves

    S1, S2 heard, no murmurs

Extremites:

    No swelling noted

    Normal muscle tone noted in all extremities

    Normal power observed in all extremities

    Deep tendon reflexes within normal limits

Differential Diagnosis

1. _____   3. _____

2. _____   4. _____

Follow-Up

1. _____   4. _____

2. _____   5. _____

3. _____

See Section III for differential diagnosis, appropriate follow-up, and brief case review.

CASE 43

A 49-year-old male is brought to the clinic by his wife. He has had a cough for the past 8 weeks.

The patient has been reluctant to be seen by his doctor for fear that it is "something really serious." His cough is productive of whitish sputum and is occasionally streaked with bright red blood. Three days ago he developed a pain in the left side of his chest. He states that the pain is very severe when he coughs, but otherwise does not bother him much. He has been feeling generally unwell for the past year and feels that his energy level has decreased significantly. His appetite is poor and he reports that he has not been sleeping well. He has noticed that his clothes seem looser over the past 2 months and thinks that he has had some weight loss, but is unsure how much. He wakes up in the middle of the night with aches and pains in his arms and his legs. He has been well in the past and has had no significant medical illnesses. He smokes a pack of cigarettes a day, which he has been doing since he was 14 years old. He drinks occasionally at present and admits to having been a heavy drinker in his teens and his twenties.

Patient History Checklist

- ☐ Patient's name
- ☐ Patient's age
- ☐ Patient's address
- ☐ Patient's occupation
- ☐ Patient's presenting complaint
- ☐ Duration of symptoms
- ☐ Presence of cough (productive/nonproductive)
- ☐ Appearance of the sputum
- ☐ Presence of blood in the sputum
- ☐ Shortness of breath
- ☐ Presence of fever

- ☐ Presence of rhinorrhea
- ☐ Presence of chest pain
- ☐ History of the pain
    - ☐ Site
    - ☐ Onset
    - ☐ Duration
    - ☐ Intensity
    - ☐ Radiation
    - ☐ Character
    - ☐ Exacerbating factors
    - ☐ Relieving factors
- ☐ History of weight loss
- ☐ Amount of weight loss
- ☐ Time period of weight loss
- ☐ Presence of night sweats
- ☐ Medical history
- ☐ Hospital admissions
- ☐ Surgical history
- ☐ Medications
- ☐ Family history
    - ☐ Cancer
    - ☐ Heart disease
    - ☐ Diabetes
    - ☐ Thyroid disease
    - ☐ Asthma/allergies
    - ☐ Others
- ☐ Social history
    - ☐ Smoking
    - ☐ Alcohol
    - ☐ Other drug use

Differential Diagnosis

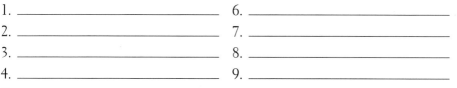

1. _____   6. _____
2. _____   7. _____
3. _____   8. _____
4. _____   9. _____
5. _____

Physical Examination Checklist

- ☐ Overall assessment
- ☐ Vitals
  - ☐ Temperature
  - ☐ Pulse—assess for tachycardia
  - ☐ Blood pressure
  - ☐ Respirations—assess for tachypnea
- ☐ Examine the face—assess mucus membranes for the presence of cyanosis
- ☐ Examine the neck
  - ☐ Assess for lymphadenopathy
  - ☐ Assess for use of accessory muscles
  - ☐ Assess the position of the trachea
- ☐ Examine the extremities
  - ☐ Assess for clubbing
  - ☐ Assess for cyanosis
- ☐ Respiratory system—examine the thorax
  - ☐ Inspect
    - ☐ Size
    - ☐ Shape
    - ☐ Symmetry
    - ☐ Movement
    - ☐ Deformities of the ribs
    - ☐ Deformities of the spine
    - ☐ Scars
  - ☐ Palpate
    - ☐ Tenderness
    - ☐ Excursion
    - ☐ Tactile fremitus
    - ☐ Chest dimensions
    - ☐ Position of the diaphragm
  - ☐ Percuss
    - ☐ All areas comparing side to side
    - ☐ Diaphragm excursion (left)
    - ☐ Diaphragm excursion (right)
  - ☐ Auscultate
    - ☐ All areas comparing side to side
    - ☐ Breath sounds

☐ Vocal resonance
☐ Whispering pectoriloquy
☐ Aegophony

Physical Examination Findings

General: 49-year-old male, anxious appearing

Vitals:

Pulse—80/minute   Temperature—97.7°F

BP—128/78 mm Hg   Respirations—16/minute

HEENT: Mouth—mucous membranes moist; no cyanosis noted

Neck:

No lymphadenopathy

No use of accessory muscles of respirations

Trachea midline

Extremities: No clubbing or cyanosis noted

Respiratory system:

Thorax normal size and shape

No asymmetry noted

No scars or deformities noted

No tenderness to palpation

Tactile fremitus increased at left base

No increased anteroposterior diameter

Dull to percussion at left base

Level of the diaphragms equal bilaterally

Decreased breath sounds noted at left base

No wheezing noted

Increased vocal resonance at left base

Whispering pectoriloquy present at left base

Aegophony noted at left base

Differential Diagnosis

1. _____   3. _____
2. _____   4. _____

Follow-Up

1. _____   4. _____
2. _____   5. _____
3. _____

See Section III for differential diagnosis, appropriate follow-up, and brief case review.

CASE 44

A 17-year-old female is seen in the emergency department complaining of fever and headache.

The patient is brought to the emergency department by her parents. She has been feeling unwell for the past 2 days with some nausea, vomiting, and fatigue. Early this morning she woke up with a severe headache and a fever. She has been febrile all day with a maximum temperature of 102°F. She has continued to feel nauseous throughout the day and has had no appetite. She also reports that she has been having some pain and difficulty moving her neck since the onset of the headache. She has had no ill contacts that she is aware of. Her parents have noticed that throughout the day she has been becoming increasingly irritable. She has been healthy in the past with no prior admissions to the hospital. She denies the presence of any other symptoms.

Patient History Checklist

☐ Patient's name
☐ Patient's age
☐ Patient's address
☐ Patient's occupation
☐ Patient's presenting complaint
☐ Presence of fever (maximum temperature)
☐ Absence/presence pain
☐ History of the pain
  ☐ Site
  ☐ Onset
  ☐ Duration
  ☐ Intensity
  ☐ Radiation
  ☐ Character
  ☐ Exacerbating factors

    ☐ Relieving factors
    ☐ Medications used to relieve symptoms
☐ Presence of dizziness
☐ Presence of nausea/vomiting
☐ Presence of fatigue
☐ Presence of irritability
☐ Presence of photophobia
☐ Difficulty concentrating
☐ Difficulty sleeping
☐ Previous episode of symptoms
☐ Presence of any skin rash
☐ Ill contacts
☐ Medications taken for the symptoms
☐ History of trauma
☐ Medical history
☐ Hospital admissions
☐ Surgical history
☐ Medications
☐ Family history
    ☐ Heart disease
    ☐ Diabetes
    ☐ Thyroid disease
    ☐ Cancer
    ☐ Others
☐ Social history
    ☐ Smoking
    ☐ Alcohol
    ☐ Other drug use

Differential Diagnosis

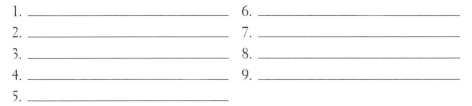

1. _____   6. _____
2. _____   7. _____
3. _____   8. _____
4. _____   9. _____
5. _____

Physical Examination Checklist

- ☐ Overall assessment
- ☐ Vitals
  - ☐ Temperature—assess for fever
  - ☐ Pulse—assess for tachycardia or bradycardia
  - ☐ Blood pressure
  - ☐ Respirations
- ☐ Evaluate mental status
  - ☐ Orientation to person, place, and time
  - ☐ Level of consciousness
  - ☐ Short-term memory
  - ☐ Long-term memory
  - ☐ Observe the patient's gait and speech
- ☐ Examine the skin
  - ☐ Rashes
  - ☐ Ecchymoses
- ☐ Examine the head—assess for masses, ecchymosis, lacerations, tenderness
- ☐ Examine the eyes—assess for papilledema
- ☐ Examine the ears
  - ☐ Assess the external ear canal for fluid drainage
  - ☐ Assess the tympanic membranes
- ☐ Assess for cervical rigidity
- ☐ Brudzinski's sign
- ☐ Kernig's sign
- ☐ Examine all cranial nerves (I–XII)

Physical Examination Findings

General: 17 year-old-female, ill appearing, patient appeared agitated throughout interview

Vitals:

Pulse—112/minute   Temperature—102.5°F

BP—94/68 mm Hg   Respirations—18/minute

Mental status:

    Patient oriented to person

    Not oriented to place or time

    Long-term memory intact

    Short-term memory impaired

    No abnormal gait observed

    Speech appropriate

Skin:

    No rashes noted

    No ecchymoses noted

HEENT:

    Head—No masses, ecchymosis, lacerations, or tenderness appreciated

    Eyes—No papilledema noted on fundoscopy

    Ears—No drainage noted; tympanic membranes visualized bilaterally

    Cervical rigidity appreciated

    Brudzinski's sign positive

    Kernig's sign positive

Cranial nerves: I–XII intact

Differential Diagnosis

1. _____   3. _____

2. _____   4. _____

Follow-Up

1. _____   4. _____

2. _____   5. _____

3. _____

See Section III for differential diagnosis, appropriate follow-up, and brief case review.

CASE 45

A 27-year-old male is seen by his primary care physician. He has vague symptoms and has generally not been feeling well for the past 3 weeks.

The patient states that he has "not been feeling himself" for the past 3 weeks. He has no interest in his usual activities. He is usually an avid baseball player, but has not been motivated to play lately. He is employed as a bank teller and usually really enjoys his job, but over the last 3 weeks has called in sick to his work seven times because he states that he just wasn't in the mood to work. He reports that he has been losing some weight, his appetite is poor, and he is not sleeping well. He finds that he is able to fall asleep at night with no problem. However, he wakes up around 3:00 in the morning and is unable to fall back asleep. He recently broke up with his long-term girlfriend and when questioned about this he states, "She's probably better off; I'm not good enough for her anyway." He has one brother with a history of depression. The rest of his family history is unremarkable. His medical history is also unremarkable.

Patient History Checklist

- ☐ Patient's name
- ☐ Patient's age
- ☐ Patient's address
- ☐ Patient's occupation
- ☐ Patient's presenting complaint
- ☐ Duration of symptoms
- ☐ Presence of fatigue
- ☐ Presence of irritability
- ☐ Difficulty concentrating
- ☐ Difficulty sleeping
- ☐ Presence of early morning waking

- ☐ Loss of appetite
- ☐ Presence of weight loss/gain
- ☐ Amount of weight loss/weight gain
- ☐ Time period of weight loss/weight gain
- ☐ Loss of interest in sexual intercourse
- ☐ Loss of interest in hobbies
- ☐ Tearfulness
- ☐ Feelings of worthlessness
- ☐ Presence of hallucinations
- ☐ Presence of delusions
- ☐ Suicidal ideation
  - ☐ Suicide plan
  - ☐ Previous suicide attempts
- ☐ Previous episode of symptoms
- ☐ Medical history
- ☐ Hospital admissions
- ☐ Surgical history
- ☐ Medications
- ☐ Family history
  - ☐ Depression
  - ☐ Psychiatric illnesses
  - ☐ Heart disease
  - ☐ Diabetes
  - ☐ Thyroid disease
  - ☐ Cancer
  - ☐ Others
- ☐ Social history
  - ☐ Smoking
  - ☐ Alcohol
  - ☐ Other drug use
  - ☐ Family situation
  - ☐ Work situation
  - ☐ Ability to function at work
  - ☐ Ability to function at home
  - ☐ Presence of support system

Differential Diagnosis

1. _____
2. _____
3. _____
4. _____
5. _____

6. _____
7. _____
8. _____
9. _____

Physical Examination Checklist

If time permits, perform an assessment for hypothyroidism. Also perform a full central nervous system examination.

Follow-Up

1. _____
2. _____
3. _____

4. _____
5. _____

See Section III for differential diagnosis, appropriate follow-up, and brief case review.

CASE 46

A 42-year-old male is seen in the clinic complaining of a burning pain in his abdomen.

The patient reports that he has been having the pain for the past 3 months. The pain comes on gradually about 1 hour following a meal. The pain is associated with nausea most of the time and on quite a few occasions he has vomited while experiencing the pain. He states that although it is unpleasant to vomit, his pain is greatly relieved by vomiting. He reports that he has noticed a significant weight loss over the past 3 months and attributes this to the fact that he now avoids a lot of his favorite foods as they seem to make the pain worse. His favorite foods are hot wings and spicy curries. His medical history is unremarkable. He denies the use of cigarettes but does admit that he drinks a 6-pack of beer a day after work. His family history is significant for alcohol abuse by both his father and one of his brothers.

Patient History Checklist

☐ Patient's name
☐ Patient's age
☐ Patient's address
☐ Patient's occupation
☐ Patient's presenting complaint
☐ Absence/presence of abdominal pain
☐ History of the pain
    ☐ Site
    ☐ Onset
    ☐ Duration
    ☐ Intensity
    ☐ Radiation
    ☐ Character

     ☐ Exacerbating factors
     ☐ Relieving factors
     ☐ Medications used to try to relieve the pain
☐ Presence of weight loss/gain
☐ Amount of weight loss/weight gain
☐ Time period of weight loss/weight gain
☐ Changes in bowel movements
☐ Changes in appetite (increased/decreased)
☐ Presence of melena
☐ Presence of hematemesis
☐ Medical history
☐ Hospital admissions
☐ Surgical history
☐ Medications
☐ Family history
     ☐ Gastric ulcers
     ☐ Heart disease
     ☐ Diabetes
     ☐ Thyroid disease
     ☐ Cancer
     ☐ Others
☐ Social history
     ☐ Smoking
     ☐ Alcohol (CAGE questions)
     ☐ Other drug use

Differential Diagnosis

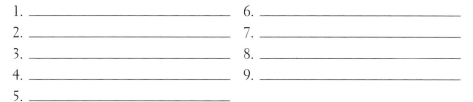

1. _____   6. _____
2. _____   7. _____
3. _____   8. _____
4. _____   9. _____
5. _____

Physical Examination Checklist

☐ Overall assessment
☐ Vitals
    ☐ Temperature
    ☐ Pulse—assess for tachycardia
    ☐ Blood pressure—assess for hypotension
    ☐ Respirations
☐ Examine the abdomen
    ☐ Inspect
    ☐ Auscultate
    ☐ Light palpation
    ☐ Deep palpation
    ☐ Assess for organomegaly (palpation and percussion)
    ☐ Assess for muscular rigidity
    ☐ Assess for rebound tenderness
☐ Perform a full cardiovascular examination, if time permits
☐ Indicate to the patient that you would like to perform a digital rectal examination, but will not do so during this examination

Physical Examination Findings

General: 42-year-old male, no acute distress
Vitals:

    Pulse—68/minute   Temperature—97.2°F
    BP—120/80 mm Hg   Respirations—12/minute

Abdomen:

    No ecchymosis visible
    No visible masses
    No striae noted
    No visible peristalsis
    Bowel sounds present in all quadrants
    No bruits heard
    No friction rubs over the spleen or liver

No tenderness to palpation
No hepatosplenomegaly
No rebound tenderness noted

Differential Diagnosis

1. _____   3. _____
2. _____   4. _____

Follow-Up

1. _____   4. _____
2. _____   5. _____
3. _____

See Section III for differential diagnosis, appropriate follow-up, and brief case review.

CASE 47

A 17-year-old male is brought to the outpatient department by his mother. He has been feeling unwell for the past week. He has had a fever and a sore throat.

The patient also complains that he has been feeling very tired over the past few days. He has not attended school since the onset of his symptoms. He has also noticed that he has some discomfort in his neck and can feel some "swollen glands." He has not actually taken his temperature at home; however, he has been feeling intermittently hot and cold. He has had no nausea or vomiting. His mother states that she is quite concerned as he seems to have been very sluggish and sleeping a lot since the onset of the symptoms. He is usually very active and plays on a lot of sports teams at school. His girlfriend has had similar symptoms for the past 2 days and has also been off school.

Patient History Checklist

- ☐ Patient's name
- ☐ Patient's age
- ☐ Patient's address
- ☐ Patient's occupation
- ☐ Patient's presenting complaint
- ☐ Duration of symptoms
- ☐ Presence of sore throat
- ☐ Presence of fever
- ☐ Presence of fatigue
- ☐ Presence of nausea/vomiting
- ☐ Changes in appetite (increased/decreased)
- ☐ Ill contacts
- ☐ Presence of rhinorrhea
- ☐ Presence of swollen glands
- ☐ Medications used during this acute episode/effect of medications used
- ☐ Allergies

☐ Medical history
☐ Hospital admissions
☐ Surgical history
☐ Medications
☐ Family history
    ☐ Heart disease
    ☐ Diabetes
    ☐ Thyroid disease
    ☐ Cancer
    ☐ Others
☐ Social history
    ☐ Smoking
    ☐ Alcohol
    ☐ Other drug use
    ☐ Involvement in contact sports

Differential Diagnosis

1. _____   6. _____
2. _____   7. _____
3. _____   8. _____
4. _____   9. _____
5. _____

Physical Examination Checklist

☐ Overall assessment
☐ Vitals
    ☐ Temperature—assess for fever
    ☐ Pulse—assess for tachycardia
    ☐ Blood pressure
    ☐ Respirations
☐ Examine the mouth
    ☐ Assess for signs of dehydration
    ☐ Assess for areas of erythema
    ☐ Assess for exudates
    ☐ Assess for signs of infection

☐ Examine the neck—assess for lymphadenopathy
☐ Examine the abdomen
    ☐ Inspect
    ☐ Auscultate
    ☐ Light palpation
    ☐ Deep palpation
    ☐ Assess for organomegaly (palpation and percussion)

Physical Examination Findings

General: 17-year-old male, unwell appearing
Vitals:

Pulse—102/minute	Temperature—101.3°F
BP—128/88 mm Hg	Respirations—16/minute

Mouth:

Tonsillar erythema noted

White exudates noted on tonsils

Mucous membranes moist

No dental caries noted

No gingivitis noted

Neck: Bilateral lymphadenopathy noted

Abdomen:

No ecchymosis visible

No visible masses

No striae noted

No visible peristalsis

Bowel sounds present in all quadrants

No bruits heard

No friction rubs over the spleen or liver

No tenderness to palpation

No hepatosplenomegaly

Differential Diagnosis

1. _____   3. _____
2. _____   4. _____

Follow-Up

1. _____   4. _____
2. _____   5. _____
3. _____

See Section III for differential diagnosis, appropriate follow-up, and brief case review.

CASE 48

A 43-year-old female is seen in the outpatient department. She complains that she has been experiencing a strange sensation in her chest which feels like butterflies.

The patient further describes the sensation as a "flutter and bump" of her heart. She has been noticing this sensation for the past 3 months. She denies any associated shortness of breath. She also denies chest pain and diaphoresis associated with the sensation. She has not had a fever and has been feeling well with the exception of these fluttering sensations. She has had no episodes of dizziness. The patient reports that she has approximately 5–10 episodes per day and has noticed that the majority of them seem to occur while she is at work. She lives at home with her husband and their four children. She has recently started back into the workforce as a bank teller for the first time in 12 years and admits that she is finding it very stressful to return to work after so many years away from it.

Patient History Checklist

- ☐ Patient's name
- ☐ Patient's age
- ☐ Patient's address
- ☐ Patient's occupation
- ☐ Patient's presenting complaint
- ☐ Frequency of palpitations
- ☐ Associated symptoms
  - ☐ Diaphoresis
  - ☐ Shortness of breath
  - ☐ Chest pain
  - ☐ Dizziness
- ☐ Diet
- ☐ Changes in appetite
- ☐ Presence of weight loss/gain
- ☐ Amount of weight loss/weight gain

- ☐ Time period of weight loss/weight gain
- ☐ Previous episodes of palpitations
- ☐ Use of nicotine
- ☐ Use of alcohol
- ☐ Use of caffeine
- ☐ Use of diet pills
- ☐ Use of illicit drugs
- ☐ Frequency and type of exercise
- ☐ Stress at present
- ☐ Medical history
- ☐ Hospital admissions
- ☐ Surgical history
- ☐ Medications
- ☐ Family history
    - ☐ Heart disease
    - ☐ Thyroid disease
    - ☐ Diabetes
    - ☐ Cancer
    - ☐ Other

Differential Diagnosis

1. _____   6. _____
2. _____   7. _____
3. _____   8. _____
4. _____   9. _____
5. _____

Physical Examination Checklist

- ☐ Overall assessment
- ☐ Vitals
    - ☐ Temperature
    - ☐ Pulse—assess for tachycardia
    - ☐ Pulse—assess for arrhythmias
    - ☐ Blood pressure—assess for hypertension
    - ☐ Respirations

- ☐ Examine the neck
  - ☐ Examine JVP wave pattern
  - ☐ Measure the JVP
  - ☐ Assess hepatojugular reflux
  - ☐ Carotid arteries—assess for bruits
- ☐ Cardiovascular system
  - ☐ Inspect the precordium
    - ☐ Shape
    - ☐ Scars
    - ☐ Pulses
    - ☐ Apex
  - ☐ Palpate the precordium
    - ☐ Tenderness
    - ☐ Pulses
    - ☐ Apex
    - ☐ Thrills
    - ☐ Heaves
  - ☐ Percuss the heart borders
  - ☐ Auscultate with the bell
    - ☐ Aortic area
    - ☐ Pulmonic area
    - ☐ Erb's point
    - ☐ Tricuspid area
    - ☐ Apex (mitral) area
  - ☐ Auscultate with the diaphragm
    - ☐ Aortic area
    - ☐ Pulmonic area
    - ☐ Erb's point
    - ☐ Tricuspid area
    - ☐ Apex (mitral) area
  - ☐ Auscultate with the bell—patient in left lateral recumbent position
  - ☐ Auscultate with the diaphragm—patient in aortic position

Physical Examination Findings

General: 43-year-old female, no acute distress
Vitals:

Pulse—78/minute   Temperature—97.7°F
BP—124/84 mm Hg   Respirations—12/minute

Neck:

No JVP noted
No hepatojugular reflux noted
No carotid bruits appreciated

Cardiovascular system:

Precordium normal shape and size
No abnormal pulsations appreciated
Apical, suprasternal, and abdominal pulsations observed
No tenderness to palpation
Apical, suprasternal, and abdominal pulsations all palpable
No thrills or heaves
S1, S2 heard, no murmurs

Differential Diagnosis

1. _____   3. _____
2. _____   4. _____

Follow-Up

1. _____   4. _____
2. _____   5. _____
3. _____

See Section III for differential diagnosis, appropriate follow-up, and brief case review.

CASE 49

A 17-year-old female is seen in the emergency room complaining of feeling light-headed and dizzy for the past 2 days

She reports that 2 days ago at school she had become very dizzy and nauseated. She does not remember exactly what happened at school, only that she woke up lying on the floor. When she "came to" there were some students around her, but no one claimed to have seen her fall. She has a large bruise on the back of her head which is tender to touch. She also reports that over the past 2 days she has been feeling very irritable and fatigued. She denies any visual disturbances or numbness, and has no difficulty walking. She is continuing to experience dizziness and headaches. Her medical history is unremarkable.

Patient History Checklist

- ☐ Patient's name
- ☐ Patient's age
- ☐ Patient's address
- ☐ Patient's occupation
- ☐ Patient's presenting complaint
- ☐ Absence/presence pain
- ☐ History of the pain
  - ☐ Site
  - ☐ Onset
  - ☐ Duration
  - ☐ Intensity
  - ☐ Radiation
  - ☐ Character
  - ☐ Exacerbating factors
  - ☐ Relieving factors
  - ☐ Medications used to relieve symptoms

- ☐ Presence of dizziness
- ☐ Presence of nausea/vomiting
- ☐ Presence of fatigue
- ☐ Sexual history
  - ☐ Age of menarche
  - ☐ Frequency of periods
  - ☐ Last menstrual period
  - ☐ Duration of periods
  - ☐ Presence of dysmenorrhea
  - ☐ Frequency of sexual intercourse
  - ☐ History of sexually transmitted diseases
  - ☐ Presence of vaginal discharge
  - ☐ Presence of dyspareunia
  - ☐ Number of pregnancies/outcomes of pregnancies
  - ☐ Number of abortions
  - ☐ Reasons for abortions
- ☐ Presence of irritability
- ☐ Difficulty concentrating
- ☐ Difficulty sleeping
- ☐ Previous episode of symptoms
- ☐ Incontinence of urine
- ☐ Incontinence of feces
- ☐ Bite injury to tongue
- ☐ History of trauma
- ☐ Medical history
- ☐ Hospital admissions
- ☐ Surgical history
- ☐ Medications

Differential Diagnosis

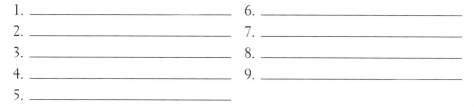

1. _____   6. _____
2. _____   7. _____
3. _____   8. _____
4. _____   9. _____
5. _____

Physical Examination Checklist

- ☐ Overall assessment
- ☐ Vitals
  - ☐ Temperature—assess for fever
  - ☐ Pulse
    - ☐ Assess for tachycardia or bradycardia
    - ☐ Assess for arrhythmias
  - ☐ Blood pressure—assess for hypotension
  - ☐ Respirations
- ☐ Evaluate mental status
  - ☐ Orientation to person, place, and time
  - ☐ Level of consciousness
  - ☐ Short-term memory
  - ☐ Long-term memory
  - ☐ Observe the patient's gait and speech
- ☐ Examine the head
  - ☐ Assess for masses, ecchymosis, lacerations, tenderness
  - ☐ Examine the tongue for bite injury
- ☐ Examine the ears
  - ☐ Assess the external ear canal for fluid drainage
  - ☐ Assess the tympanic membranes
- ☐ Examine the eyes—assess for conjunctival pallor
- ☐ Examine all cranial nerves (I–XII)
- ☐ Examine the sensory system
  - ☐ Check for pain and crude touch in all parts of the body
  - ☐ Romberg's test
  - ☐ Proprioception at fingers and toes
  - ☐ Vibratory sense
  - ☐ Stereognosis
  - ☐ Graphesthesia
  - ☐ 2-point discrimination
  - ☐ Point localization
  - ☐ Extinction
- ☐ Examine the motor system
  - ☐ Inspect the motor system for atrophy, fasciculations, and involuntary movements
  - ☐ Palpate all limbs for muscle tone

□ Check all major muscle groups for power
□ Check all reflexes
   □ Abdominal
   □ Plantar
   □ Biceps
   □ Triceps
   □ Brachioradialis
   □ Knee
   □ Ankle
□ Examine the cerebellum
   □ Ask the patient to walk in a straight line, heel to toe
   □ Ask the patient to walk in a straight line on his/her heels
   □ Ask the patient to walk in a straight line on his/her toes
   □ Ask the patient to perform the finger–nose test
   □ Ask the patient to perform the knee–heel–shin test
   □ Check for dysdiadochokinesia

Physical Examination Findings

General: 17-year-old female, no acute distress
Vitals:

Pulse—78/minute	Temperature—97.9°F
BP—110/70 mm Hg	Respirations—14/minute

Mental status:

Patient oriented to person, place, and time
Patient awake and alert
Short- and long-term memory intact
No abnormal gait observed
Speech appropriate

HEENT:

Head—No masses, ecchymosis, lacerations, or tenderness appreciated
Mouth—No bite injury to tongue
Ears—No drainage noted; tympanic membranes visualized bilaterally
Eyes—No conjunctival pallor noted

Cranial nerves: I–XII intact

Sensory system: Sensation intact bilaterally

Motor system:

    No atrophy noted

    No fasciculations

    Normal muscle tone noted in all extremities

    Normal power observed in all extremities

    Deep tendon reflexes intact

    Abdominal reflex present

    Plantar reflex down going

Cerebellum: No abnormalities noted

Differential Diagnosis

1. _____   3. _____
2. _____   4. _____

Follow-Up

1. _____   4. _____
2. _____   5. _____
3. _____

See Section III for differential diagnosis, appropriate follow-up, and brief case review.

CASE 50

A 51-year-old female is seen by her primary care physician complaining of amenorrhea.

The patient reports that she has not had her period for 7 weeks. In the past her menstrual periods have always been regular occurring every 31 days. For the past year they have not been quite as regular but have never been as late as this. She has not been sleeping well for the past 6 months and finds that she feels agitated a lot of the time. Her mother went through "the change" at age 55 and she wonders if she is going through "the change" now. She is also a little bit concerned that this really is not menopause and she is actually pregnant. She is sexually active with her husband and they do not use any form of birth control. They have two children who are both away at college. She denies any breast tenderness. She has not experienced any hot flashes.

Patient History Checklist

- ☐ Patient's name
- ☐ Patient's age
- ☐ Patient's address
- ☐ Patient's occupation
- ☐ Patient's presenting complaint
- ☐ Sexual history
    - ☐ Last menstrual period
    - ☐ Age of menarche
    - ☐ Frequency of periods
    - ☐ Duration of periods
    - ☐ Presence of vaginal discharge
    - ☐ Presence of vaginal bleeding/spotting
    - ☐ Number of pregnancies/outcomes of pregnancies
    - ☐ Number of abortions
    - ☐ Reasons for abortions

- ☐ History of sexually transmitted diseases
- ☐ Presence of dyspareunia
☐ Presence of hot flashes
☐ Presence of mood swings
☐ Presence of sleep disturbances
☐ Changes in sex drive
☐ Presence of weight gain
☐ Amount of weight gain
☐ Time period of weight gain
☐ Presence of breast tenderness
☐ Presence of breast enlargement
☐ Presence of nipple discharge
☐ Presence of morning sickness
☐ Presence of fatigue
☐ Mother's age at menopause
☐ Medical history
☐ Hospital admissions
☐ Surgical history
☐ Medications
☐ Family history
  - ☐ Breast cancer
  - ☐ Heart disease
  - ☐ Diabetes
  - ☐ Thyroid disease
  - ☐ Others
☐ Social history
  - ☐ Smoking
  - ☐ Alcohol
  - ☐ Other drug use
  - ☐ Feelings of anxiety
  - ☐ Exercise
  - ☐ Diet

Differential Diagnosis

1. _____   6. _____
2. _____   7. _____
3. _____   8. _____
4. _____   9. _____
5. _____

Physical Examination Checklist

☐ Overall assessment
☐ Vitals
   ☐ Temperature
   ☐ Pulse
   ☐ Blood pressure
   ☐ Respirations
☐ Examine the abdomen
   ☐ Inspect
   ☐ Auscultate
   ☐ Light palpation
   ☐ Deep palpation
   ☐ Assess for organomegaly (palpation and percussion)
   ☐ Assess for pelvic abdominal masses/fundal height
   ☐ Assess for fetal movements
☐ Indicate to the patient that you would like to perform a breast examination and a pelvic examination, but will not do so during this examination

Physical Examination Findings

General: 51-year-old female, no acute distress
Vitals:

Pulse—72/minute   Temperature—98.9°F
BP—142/98 mm Hg   Respirations—12/minute

Abdomen:

> No ecchymosis visible
> No visible masses
> No striae noted
> No visible peristalsis
> Bowel sounds present in all quadrants
> No bruits heard
> No friction rubs over the spleen or liver
> No tenderness to palpation
> No hepatosplenomegaly
> Fundus not palpable
> No fetal movements appreciated

Differential Diagnosis

1. _____   3. _____
2. _____   4. _____

Follow-Up

1. _____   4. _____
2. _____   5. _____
3. _____

See Section III for differential diagnosis, appropriate follow-up, and brief case review.

A 74-year-old female is seen in the clinic complaining of increasing difficulty reading.

The patient first noticed that she was having some changes in her vision about 6 months ago and since that time the problem seems to have become worse. She complains that at the onset of the symptoms she found that her vision seemed cloudy. Her vision appeared hazy. Since that time she has found that her ability to distinguish colors has worsened. She complains that the vision in her left eyes seems to be much worse than the vision in her right eye. She has been wearing reading glasses for the past 30 years and her vision has remained steady until recently. She is able to do her daily household chores without difficulty; however, finds that her night vision is affected due to the hazy appearance of objects. She also has a problem with bright lights, as they seem to cause halos around objects. Her medical history is significant for depression for which she has been treated for the past 10 years. She lives with her husband and their two cats. She denies the use of cigarettes and drinks three to four glasses of white wine a day.

Patient History Checklist

☐ Patient's name
☐ Patient's age
☐ Patient's address
☐ Patient's occupation
☐ Patient's presenting complaint
☐ Duration of symptoms
☐ Presence of headaches
☐ Presence of blurred vision
☐ Previous problems with vision
☐ Presence of cloudy vision
☐ Sensitivity to light

☐ Difficulty with night vision
☐ Presence of eye pain
☐ Dryness of the eyes
☐ Presence of dizziness
☐ Ability to perform daily activities
☐ Use of glasses
☐ Medical history
☐ Hospital admissions
☐ Surgical history
☐ Medications
☐ Family history
    ☐ Heart disease
    ☐ Diabetes
    ☐ Thyroid disease
    ☐ Cancer
    ☐ Others
☐ Social history
    ☐ Smoking
    ☐ Alcohol
    ☐ Other drug use

Differential Diagnosis

1. _____   6. _____
2. _____   7. _____
3. _____   8. _____
4. _____   9. _____
5. _____

Physical Examination Checklist

☐ Overall assessment
☐ Vitals
    ☐ Temperature
    ☐ Pulse
    ☐ Blood pressure
    ☐ Respirations

☐ Examine the eyes
  ☐ Alignment
  ☐ Lid swelling
  ☐ Lid lesions
  ☐ Lid retraction
  ☐ Check visual acuity
  ☐ Check peripheral visual fields
  ☐ Examine anterior chamber
  ☐ Examine the iris
  ☐ Examine the pupils
☐ Opthalmoscopic examination
  ☐ Obstruction to light by lens
  ☐ Retinal hemorrhages
  ☐ Microaneurysms
  ☐ Neovascularization
  ☐ Hard exudates

Physical Examination Findings

General: 74-year-old female, no acute distress
Vitals:

Pulse—82/minute   Temperature—97.9°F
BP—144/88 mm Hg   Respirations—14/minute

Eyes:

No asymmetry noted

No lid swellings, lesions, or retractions noted

Visual acuity 20/70 in left eye, 20/50 in right eye, 20/40 in both eyes

No peripheral field deficits noted

Anterior chamber clear

Pupils equal and reactive to light and accommodation bilaterally

Mild opacity of the lens noted on the left

No retinal hemorrhages, microaneurysms, neovascularization, or hard exudates noted

Differential Diagnosis

1. _____   3. _____
2. _____   4. _____

Follow-Up

1. _____   4. _____
2. _____   5. _____
3. _____

See Section III for differential diagnosis, appropriate follow-up, and brief case review.

CASE 52

A 61-year-old male is seen in the outpatient clinic. He complains that he noticed that he has some blood in his urine.

The patient has been to the bathroom twice since getting up this morning and both times noticed that there was some bright red blood in his urine. He is not experiencing any abdominal pain and does not complain that he has any pain either during urination or following urination. He has no other complaints. He denies nausea and vomiting. He has never had any previous episodes of blood in his urine. He denies frequency and urgency. He has not had a fever. He has not noticed any discharge from his penis. His medical history is only significant for recurrent episodes of gout.

Patient History Checklist

☐ Patient's name
☐ Patient's age
☐ Patient's address
☐ Patient's occupation
☐ Patient's presenting complaint
☐ Presence of blood in urine
☐ Presence of abdominal pain
☐ Presence of dysuria
☐ Presence of urgency
☐ Presence of frequency
☐ Decreased force of urinary stream
☐ Previous episodes of symptoms
☐ Presence of nausea/vomiting
☐ Presence of fatigue
☐ Presence of fever
☐ History of sexually transmitted diseases
☐ Presence of discharge from penis

☐ Number of current sexual partners
☐ History of trauma
☐ Medical history
☐ Hospital admissions
☐ Surgical history
☐ Medications
☐ Family history
    ☐ Cancer
    ☐ Heart disease
    ☐ Diabetes
    ☐ Thyroid disease
    ☐ Others
☐ Social history
    ☐ Smoking
    ☐ Alcohol
    ☐ Other drug use

Differential Diagnosis

1. _____   6. _____
2. _____   7. _____
3. _____   8. _____
4. _____   9. _____
5. _____

Physical Examination Checklist

☐ Overall assessment
☐ Vitals
    ☐ Temperature
    ☐ Pulse
    ☐ Blood pressure
    ☐ Respirations
☐ Examine the abdomen
    ☐ Inspect
    ☐ Auscultate

□ Light palpation
□ Deep palpation
□ Assess for organomegaly (palpation and percussion)
□ Indicate to the patient that you would like to perform a digital rectal examination, but will not do so during this examination
□ Indicate to the patient that you would like to examine his genitalia, but will not do so during this examination

Physical Examination Findings

General: 61-year-old male, no acute distress

Vitals:

Pulse—94/minute	Temperature—99.1°F
BP—138/90 mm Hg	Respirations—12/minute

Abdomen:

No ecchymosis visible

No visible masses

No striae noted

No visible peristalsis

Normal male hair distribution

Bowel sounds present in all quadrants

No bruits heard

No friction rubs over the spleen or liver

No tenderness to palpation

No hepatosplenomegaly

Differential Diagnosis

1. _____   3. _____

2. _____   4. _____

Follow-Up

1. _____   4. _____

2. _____   5. _____

3. _____

See Section III for differential diagnosis, appropriate follow-up, and brief case review.

CASE 53

A 16-year-old female is seen in the emergency department. She has been experiencing severe abdominal pain for the past 24 hours.

The patient has been febrile over the same period of time. The pain is localized to her pelvic region particularly on her right side. She describes the pain as a sharp pain—a 6 on a scale of 1–10, with 10 being the most severe. She has been feeling nauseated over the past 24 hours and has vomited three times. Her appetite has been very poor although she has been trying to take sips of fluids since the onset of the symptoms. She has noticed that she has been having some vaginal discharge for the past 2 weeks. The discharge is greenish in color and has a foul odor. She has not experienced any dysuria. She is sexually active with one partner and denies ever having any sexually transmitted diseases in the past. She is taking oral contraceptives and admits that she and her partner do not take any precautions against sexually transmitted diseases.

Patient History Checklist

- ☐ Patient's name
- ☐ Patient's age
- ☐ Patient's address
- ☐ Patient's occupation
- ☐ Patient's presenting complaint
- ☐ Sexual history
  - ☐ Age of menarche
  - ☐ Frequency of periods
  - ☐ Last menstrual period
  - ☐ Duration of periods
  - ☐ Presence of dysmenorrhea
  - ☐ Frequency of sexual intercourse
  - ☐ Interest in sexual intercourse

- ☐ Age at first sexual intercourse
- ☐ Number of sexual partners (past and present)
- ☐ Method of birth control
- ☐ Use of condoms
- ☐ History of sexually transmitted diseases
- ☐ Presence of vaginal discharge
- ☐ Presence of dyspareunia
- ☐ Number of pregnancies/outcomes of pregnancies
- ☐ Number of abortions
- ☐ Reasons for abortions
- ☐ Presence of weight loss/gain
- ☐ Amount of weight loss/weight gain
- ☐ Time period of weight loss/weight gain
- ☐ Partner's details
  - ☐ Age
  - ☐ Occupation
  - ☐ History of sexually transmitted diseases
  - ☐ Number of sexual partners
  - ☐ Number of children, if any
- ☐ Medical history
- ☐ Hospital admissions
- ☐ Surgical history
- ☐ Medications
- ☐ Family history
  - ☐ Heart disease
  - ☐ Diabetes
  - ☐ Hypertension
  - ☐ Cancer
  - ☐ Others
- ☐ Social history
  - ☐ Smoking
  - ☐ Alcohol
  - ☐ Other drug use
  - ☐ Family situation

Differential Diagnosis

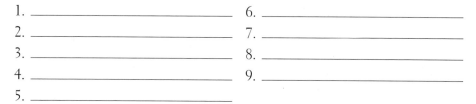

Physical Examination Checklist

- ☐ Overall assessment
- ☐ Vitals
  - ☐ Temperature—assess for fever
  - ☐ Pulse—assess for tachycardia
  - ☐ Blood pressure—assess for hypotension
  - ☐ Respirations
- ☐ Examine the abdomen
  - ☐ Inspect
  - ☐ Auscultate
  - ☐ Light palpation
  - ☐ Deep palpation
  - ☐ Assess for organomegaly (palpation and percussion)
  - ☐ Assess for CVA tenderness
  - ☐ Assess for muscular rigidity
  - ☐ Assess for referred rebound tenderness
  - ☐ Assess for rebound tenderness
  - ☐ Rovsing's sign
  - ☐ Psoas sign
  - ☐ Obturator sign
  - ☐ Cutaneous hyperesthesia
- ☐ Indicate to the patient that you would like to perform a pelvic examination including vaginal cultures, but will not do so during this examination

Physical Examination Findings

General: 16-year-old female, anxious appearing
Vitals:

Pulse — 88/minute   Temperature — 99.4°F
BP — 132/86 mm Hg   Respirations — 14/minute

Abdomen:

No ecchymosis visible
No visible masses
No striae noted
No visible peristalsis
Bowel sounds present in all quadrants
No bruits heard
No friction rubs over the spleen or liver
Tenderness to palpation in pelvic region
Tenderness to palpation in the right lower quadrant
No hepatosplenomegaly
No CVA tenderness
No referred rebound tenderness noted
No rebound tenderness noted
Rovsing's sign negative
Psoas sign negative
Obturator sign negative
No cutaneous hyperesthesia noted

Differential Diagnosis

1. _____   3. _____
2. _____   4. _____

Follow-Up

1. _____   4. _____

2. _____   5. _____

3. _____

See Section III for differential diagnosis, appropriate follow-up, and brief case review.

CASE 54

A 52-year-old male is seen in the clinic. He complains that he has been feeling very tired lately and is concerned about the control of his diabetes.

He has been diabetic for the past 5 years. He checks his blood glucose twice a day and the usual range is 100–250 mmol/dL. On further questioning he admits that he has been feeling depressed lately because he has been unable to have intercourse with his wife. It has been several months since he has been able to sustain an erection and he has not managed to have penetrative intercourse with his wife for the past 5–6 months. He states that he still desires intercourse with his wife and feels that his increasing anxiety regarding this problem is probably contributing to making the problem worse. He has also noticed that upon waking up in the morning he no longer has morning erections.

Patient History Checklist

☐ Patient's name
☐ Patient's age
☐ Patient's address
☐ Patient's occupation
☐ Patient's presenting complaint
☐ Presence of fatigue
☐ Presence of irritability
☐ Difficulty concentrating
☐ Difficulty sleeping
☐ Presence of early morning waking
☐ Loss of appetite
☐ Presence of weight loss/gain
☐ Amount of weight loss/weight gain
☐ Time period of weight loss/weight gain
☐ Loss of interest in sexual intercourse with wife or with other partners, if applicable

- ☐ Date of last successful intercourse
- ☐ Ability to have intercourse with partners other than wife (if relevant)
- ☐ Absence of morning erections
- ☐ History of sexually transmitted diseases
- ☐ Loss of interest in hobbies
- ☐ Tearfulness
- ☐ Suicidal ideation
- ☐ Previous episode of symptoms
- ☐ Medical history
- ☐ Hospital admissions
- ☐ Surgical history
- ☐ Medications (especially antihypertensives and diabetic drugs)
  - ☐ Family history
  - ☐ Depression
  - ☐ Psychiatric illnesses
  - ☐ Heart disease
  - ☐ Diabetes
  - ☐ Thyroid disease
  - ☐ Cancer
  - ☐ Others
- ☐ Social history
  - ☐ Smoking
  - ☐ Alcohol
  - ☐ Other drug use
  - ☐ Family situation
  - ☐ Wife's reaction to impotency

Differential Diagnosis

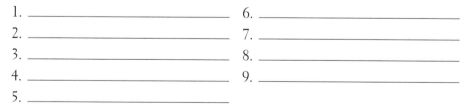

1. _____   6. _____
2. _____   7. _____
3. _____   8. _____
4. _____   9. _____
5. _____

Physical Examination Checklist

☐ If a physical examination is required, perform an assessment of the patient's
   diabetes
☐ Indicate to the patient that you would like to examine his genitalia, but will
   not do so during this examination

Follow-Up

1. _____   4. _____

2. _____   5. _____

3. _____

See Section III for differential diagnosis, appropriate follow-up, and brief case
review.

CASE 55

A 22-year-old female is seen in the outpatient clinic complaining of abdominal pain.

The pain started 24 hours ago and is becoming progressively worse. She has not noticed any aggravating or relieving factors. The pain is located in the left lower quadrant and does not radiate. She rates the pain as an 8 on a scale of 1–10, with 10 being the worst pain. She denies vaginal discharge. She has not had any episodes of diarrhea or constipation and has not experienced any nausea or vomiting. Her appetite has been poor since the onset of the pain and she has been unable to sleep. She lives with her boyfriend and is employed in a restaurant as a waitress. Her last menstrual period was 5 weeks ago, but the patient states that her periods are often irregular. She is sexually active and uses condoms as a method of birth control. She has never been pregnant in the past and denies ever having any sexually transmitted diseases.

Patient History Checklist

☐ Patient's name
☐ Patient's age
☐ Patient's address
☐ Patient's occupation
☐ Patient's presenting complaint
☐ Absence/presence of abdominal pain
☐ History of the pain
    ☐ Site
    ☐ Onset
    ☐ Duration
    ☐ Intensity
    ☐ Radiation
    ☐ Character

- ☐ Exacerbating factors
- ☐ Relieving factors
- ☐ Changes in bowel movements
- ☐ Changes in appetite (increased/decreased)
- ☐ Presence of nausea/vomiting
- ☐ Changes in menstrual cycle
- ☐ Frequency of micturition
- ☐ Presence of dysuria
- ☐ Presence of nocturia
- ☐ Presence of hematuria
- ☐ Sexual history
  - ☐ Age of menarche
  - ☐ Frequency of periods
  - ☐ Last menstrual period
  - ☐ Duration of periods
  - ☐ Presence of dysmenorrhea
  - ☐ Frequency of sexual intercourse
  - ☐ Number of sexual partners
  - ☐ History of sexually transmitted diseases
  - ☐ Date of last pelvic examination
  - ☐ Results of last pelvic examination
  - ☐ Presence of vaginal discharge
  - ☐ Presence of dyspareunia
  - ☐ Number of pregnancies/outcomes of pregnancies
  - ☐ Number of abortions
  - ☐ Reasons for abortions
- ☐ Presence of weight loss/gain
- ☐ Amount of weight loss/weight gain
- ☐ Time period of weight loss/weight gain
- ☐ Changes in breasts
- ☐ Changes in skin pigmentation
- ☐ Partner's details
  - ☐ Age
  - ☐ Occupation
  - ☐ History of sexually transmitted diseases
  - ☐ Number of sexual partners
  - ☐ Number of children, if any

- ☐ Medical history
- ☐ Hospital admissions
- ☐ Surgical history
- ☐ Medications
- ☐ Family history
    - ☐ Heart disease
    - ☐ Diabetes
    - ☐ Hypertension
    - ☐ Cancer
    - ☐ Others
- ☐ Social history
    - ☐ Smoking
    - ☐ Alcohol
    - ☐ Other drug use
    - ☐ Family situation

Differential Diagnosis

1. _____   6. _____
2. _____   7. _____
3. _____   8. _____
4. _____   9. _____
5. _____

Physical Examination Checklist

- ☐ Overall assessment
- ☐ Vitals
    - ☐ Temperature—assess for fever
    - ☐ Pulse—assess for tachycardia or bradycardia
    - ☐ Blood pressure—assess for hypotension
    - ☐ Respirations
- ☐ Examine the eyes—assess for conjunctival pallor
- ☐ Examine the mouth—assess for signs of dehydration
- ☐ Examine the abdomen

☐ Inspect
☐ Auscultate
☐ Light palpation
☐ Deep palpation
☐ Assess for organomegaly (palpation and percussion)
☐ Assess for CVA tenderness
☐ Assess for muscular rigidity
☐ Assess for referred rebound tenderness
☐ Assess for rebound tenderness
☐ Rovsing's sign
☐ Psoas sign
☐ Obturator sign
☐ Cutaneous hyperesthesia
☐ Indicate to the patient that you would like to perform a pelvic examination including vaginal cultures, but will not do so during this examination

Physical Examination Findings

General: 22-year-old female, uncomfortable appearing

Vitals:

Pulse—102/minute	Temperature—99.2°F
BP—138/88 mm Hg	Respirations—18/minute

HEENT:

Eyes—No conjunctival pallor noted

Mouth—No crackes/fissures noted; mucous membranes moist

Abdomen:

No ecchymosis visible

No visible masses

No striae noted

No visible peristalsis

Bowel sounds present in all quadrants

No bruits heard

No friction rubs over the spleen or liver

Marked tenderness to palpation in the left lower quadrant
Some guarding noted
No hepatosplenomegaly
No CVA tenderness
No referred rebound tenderness noted
No rebound tenderness noted
Rovsing's sign negative
Psoas sign negative
Obturator sign negative
No cutaneous hyperesthesia noted

Differential Diagnosis

1. _____   3. _____
2. _____   4. _____

Follow-Up

1. _____   4. _____
2. _____   5. _____
3. _____

See Section III for differential diagnosis and appropriate follow-up.

Case Answers: Differential Diagnosis and Brief Case Review

CASE 1

Differential Diagnosis

1. *Transient ischemic attack*
2. Cerebral vascular accident
3. Multiple cerebral emboli
4. Subacute bacterial endocarditis
5. Hypoglycemia
6. Central nervous system mass/tumor
7. Cerebral abscess
8. Subdural hematoma
9. Drug use/abuse
10. Seizure disorder

Follow-Up

1. Computed tomography (CT) scan
2. Electroencephalogram (EEG)
3. Fasting blood glucose
4. Electrocardiogram (ECG)
5. Doppler angiogram of carotid vessels
6. Echocardiogram (EcHO)
7. Toxicology (drug screening)

Brief Case Review

Risk factors for a TIA include hypertension, diabetes, hypercholesterolemia, obesity, smoking, and a family history of heart disease and stroke. The patient in this case has quite a few risk factors for TIA including a history of smoking, two previous heart attacks, and hypertension. The symptoms of a TIA include numbness and paralysis particularly affecting one side of the body, difficulty with speech, dizziness, blindness, or blurred vision affecting one or both eyes. The symptoms of a TIA resolve within 24 hours as opposed to the symptoms of a stroke, which may be permanent.

CASE 2

Differential Diagnosis

1. *Bipolar disorder*
2. Schizophrenia
3. Brief psychotic disorder
4. Schizophreniform disorder
5. Schizoaffective disorder
6. Drug abuse

Follow-Up

Toxicology (drug screening)

Brief Case Review

The most likely diagnosis in this case is bipolar disorder, given the history of depressed episodes along with the patient's current behavior. During a manic episode, patients often exhibit increased energy, euphoria, irritability, insomnia, increased sexual drive, poor judgment, and drug/alcohol abuse. During a depressed episode the patient can exhibit all the symptoms of depression (see also Brief Case Review for Case 45). An important aspect of the patient interview is to assess patient safety. The patient's current living situation should also be assessed. Psychotherapy should be recommended.

CASE 3

Differential Diagnosis

1. *Achalasia*
2. Goiter
3. Abnormal relaxation of the upper esophageal sphincter
4. Esophageal webs
5. Scleroderma
6. Chagas' disease
7. Globus hystericus
8. Esophageal carcinoma

Follow-Up

1. Digital rectal examination (DRE)
2. Stool guiac
3. Thyroid stimulating hormone (TSH)
4. Free thyroxine (T4)/free triiodothyroxine (T3)
5. Complete blood count (CBC)
6. Barium swallow
7. Esophagogastroduodenoscopy (EGD)

Brief Case Review

Achalasia is due to a motor disturbance of the lower esophagus and failure of the esophageal sphincter to open properly. Patients with achalasia experience difficulty with both liquids and solids. There are many other causes of dysphagia to consider in this case. Important aspects of the history include in particular, what foods the patient is having difficulty with, solids, liquids, or both. Also important is to ascertain whether there has been a change in the symptoms since the onset, for example, difficulty swallowing only liquids at the onset progressing to difficulty swallowing both liquids and solids. A travel history should be included since Chagas' disease is also a cause of dysphagia. Complete and thorough examination of the thyroid gland is a vital part of the physical examination as an enlarged gland may be the underlying cause of the dysphagia. CBC and stool guiac are useful to assess for any GI bleeding. During the interview, the patient should be educated regarding diet and healthy lifestyle choices.

CASE 4

Differential Diagnosis

Hip pain

1. *Hip fracture*
2. Trauma
3. Bursitis
4. Osteoarthritis

Fall

1. *Cardiac arrhythmia*
2. Postural hypotension
3. Anemia

Follow-Up

1. Hip X-ray
2. Orthostatic blood pressures
3. Electrocardiogram (ECG)
4. Complete blood count (CBC)

Brief Case Review

Common complaints of patients who have sustained a hip fracture include pain and inability to bear weight. Physical examination may reveal bruising over the hip area, pain on palpation of the affected hip, limited active and passive movement, as well as a shortened externally rotated limb. Important diagnosis and follow-up to be considered in this case is not only the resulting injury from the fall but also the reason for the fall. This patient should be assessed for cardiac arrhythmias, postural hypotension, and causes of postural hypotension such as anemia. In the case presented, the patient resides in an assisted living situation. Were this not the case, careful evaluation of the patients home situation as well as her ability to care for herself or the presence of a care giver following return home should be evaluated.

CASE 5

Differential Diagnosis

1. *Peripheral vascular disease*
2. Trauma
3. Buerger's disease
4. Lumbar disc degeneration
5. Abdominal aneurysm
6. Cardiac disease and systemic embolism

Follow-Up

1. Doppler ultrasound of the lower limb arteries
2. Electrocardiogram (ECG)
3. Ankle-brachial index (ABI)
4. X-ray of the lumbar spine
5. Lipid profile
6. Fasting blood glucose

Brief Case Review

Remember the five Ps of arterial insufficiency: pallor, pain, paresthesias, pulse-lessness, and perishingly cold. The most common complaint with peripheral vascular disease is intermittent claudication, which is pain upon exercise which subsides with rest. Doppler ultrasound will help to determine the blood flow to the lower extremities. A lipid profile should be done as hypercholesterolemia is often an underlying factor for peripheral vascular disease. Other causes of the symptoms to consider are disc degeneration, which can be assessed by X-ray of the lower back, and diabetes (peripheral neuropathy), which can be assessed by checking a fasting blood glucose level. Every effort to help the patient to stop smoking should be made.

CASE 6

Differential Diagnosis

1. *Congestive heart failure*
2. Cardiac arrhythmia
3. Pneumonia
4. Asthma
5. Anemia

Follow-Up

1. Chest X-ray (CXR)
2. Electrocardiogram (ECG)
3. Cardiac enzymes (CK, CK-MB, Troponin)
4. Echocardiogram (EcHO)
5. Stress test
6. Lipid profile
7. Pulmonary function tests (PFTs)
8. Arterial blood gases (ABGs)
9. Complete blood count (CBC)

Brief Case Review

Common symptoms of congestive heart failure include shortness of breath, cough, often productive of pink frothy sputum, weakness, and fatigue. Patients also commonly complain of paroxysmal nocturnal dyspnea and often report that they either sleep with many pillows or that they sleep upright in a recliner. The most common causes of CHF are hypertension, valve disease, ischemic heart disease, and diseases of the myocardium itself. Left heart failure often leads to right heart failure and the patient may notice pitting edema of the lower extremities and a tender enlarged liver may be present. An ECG should be performed to rule out a cardiac arrhythmia. Primary respiratory causes of dyspnea should also be ruled out. A CBC should be done to rule out anemia.

CASE 7

Differential Diagnosis

1. *Cerumen impaction*
2. Otitis media
3. Labyrinthitis
4. Sinus infection
5. Meniere's disease

Follow-Up

Irrigation of affected ear

Brief Case Review

The follow-up in a case such as this one is going to be based almost exclusively on the physical examination findings. In this case, the cause of decreased hearing is impacted cerumen. This is a very common cause of hearing loss. In the case of a patient in whom both tympanic membranes are visualized and there does not seem to be any impacted cerumen there is a need for an extensive follow-up in order to make a diagnosis. The follow-up may include audiometry, CT scan of the head, tympanometry, and caloric test based on the physical examination findings.

CASE 8

Differential Diagnosis

1. *Pancreatitis*
2. Cholecystitis
3. Gastroesophageal reflux
4. Alcoholic gastritis
5. Hepatitis
6. Esophageal spasm

Follow-Up

1. Digital rectal examination (DRE)
2. Amylase level
3. Lipase level
4. Stool guiac
5. Complete blood count (CBC)
6. Liver function tests (LFTs)
7. Abdominal ultrasound

Brief Case Review

The most common cause of acute pancreatitis is alcohol abuse. A thorough history of the patient's alcohol use should be ascertained. Other causes of pancreatitis include cholelithiasis, certain medications, hypertriglyceridemia, pancreatic carcinoma, and peptic ulcer disease. The common symptoms of pancreatitis include epigastric pain (usually severe) radiating to the back, nausea, vomiting, and fever. Tachycardia, tachypnea, and hypotension may all be present. In some cases Grey Turner sign and/or Cullen sign may be present.

CASE 9

Differential Diagnosis

1. *Pneumothorax*
2. Pneumonia
3. Myocardial infarction
4. Pulmonary infarct
5. Lung abscess
6. Bronchitis
7. Congestive heart failure
8. Bronchospasm

Follow-Up

1. Chest X-ray (CXR)
2. Arterial blood gases (ABGs)
3. Echocardiogram (EcHO)

Brief Case Review

Common symptoms of a pneumothorax include chest pain (usually sharp, stabbing in nature), shortness of breath, and fatigue. The patient may also experience tachycardia and hypotension. There are numerous causes of pneumothorax. These causes include trauma, underlying lung disease such as asthma, whooping cough, and tuberculosis. On occasion there may not be an obvious predisposing factor and the cause may remain unknown. A CXR is a very important diagnosis test in this case as it will help to differentiate between pneumothorax, pneumonia, and congestive heart failure. These patients often require the placement of a chest tube.

CASE 10

Differential Diagnosis

1. *Cholecystitis*
2. Pancreatitis
3. Gastroesophageal reflux
4. Alcoholic gastritis
5. Hepatitis
6. Esophageal spasm
7. Appendicitis

Follow-Up

1. Digital rectal examination (DRE)
2. Ultrasound
3. Endoscopic retrograde cholangiopancreatography (ERCP)
4. Lipid profile
5. Serum amylase
6. Serum lipase

Brief Case Review

The common symptoms of cholecystitis include abdominal pain generally col-
icky in nature located in the right upper quadrant. Nausea, vomiting, and fever
may also occur. Women are more commonly affected compared to men. The
pain may be noted to follow a fatty meal. Ninety percent of cases are caused by
gallstones in the gallbladder. The common bile duct may become blocked as
the result of a passing stone and give rise to changes in both the color of the urine

and the stool and jaundice may occur. Ultrasound is a useful diagnostic tool. Lipid profile is also important in this case as part of the follow-up since most gallstones are cholesterol stones as opposed to the less common pigment stones. ERCP is useful for looking at the ducts and observing stones or strictures. As pancreatitis is a common complication of choledocholithiasis, serum amylase and lipase should be assessed. Remember, whenever abdominal pathology is suspected, a complete examination includes a DRE.

CASE 11

Differential Diagnosis

1. *Alzheimer's dementia*
2. Multi-infarct dementia
3. Delirium
4. Hypothyroidism
5. Depression
6. Thyroxine overuse

Follow-Up

1. Thyroid stimulating hormone (TSH)
2. Free thyroxine (T4)/free triiodothyroxine (T3)
3. Complete blood count (CBC)
4. Urinalysis (U/A)
5. Electrolytes
6. Venereal Disease Research Laboratory (VDRL)
7. Chest X-ray (CXR)
8. Electrocardiogram (ECG)

Brief Case Review

Symptoms of dementia include memory loss, particularly short-term memory, difficulty concentrating, difficulty performing every day tasks, disorientation to person, place, and time, as well as changes in mood and personality. The term dementia encompasses a lot of diseases. The most common cause of dementia is Alzheimer's disease. All possibilities of the underlying cause must be investigated, including infectious causes such as syphilis. In this case it is important to make sure that the patient's hypothyroidism is being treated appropriately. Exploration of the patients home and safety situation is extremely important. Evaluation of her support system as well as ensuring that the patient has an adequate care giver are vital components of this case.

CASE 12

Differential Diagnosis

1. Bacterial infection, including
   bacteremia
   pneumonia
   urinary tract infection (UTI)
   pyelonephritis
   otitis media
   meningitis
2. Viral infection
3. Dehydration

Follow-Up

1. Full physical examination
2. Complete blood count (CBC)
3. Blood cultures
4. Urinalysis (U/A)
5. Urine culture
6. Assessment of hydration/rehydration needs
7. Lumbar puncture (LP) (if necessary)

Brief Case Review

Fever in an infant should never be taken lightly. There are a lot of things to consider based on both the symptoms as well as the age of the infant. Obtaining information regarding the pregnancy as well as the delivery is vital to the case. Remember to find out if the mother was tested for beta hemolytic streptococci (group B strep) during the pregnancy, and if positive, was she treated during labor. Another important factor is the infant's hydration status. Inquiring about feedings (how often/how much) and the number of wet diapers can help to ascertain the hydration of the infant. The mother in this case should be encouraged to bring the infant in for an evaluation. LP should always be considered in an infant with a fever if no other cause for the fever has been identified.

CASE 13

Differential Diagnosis

1. *Schizophrenia*
2. Brief psychotic disorder
3. Drug use/abuse

4. Delusional disorder
5. Schizoaffective disorder
6. Schizophreniform disorder
7. Hypothyroidism

Follow-Up

1. Blood alcohol level
2. Toxicology (drug screening)
3. Thyroid stimulating hormone (TSH)
4. Free thyroxine (T4)/free triiodothyroxine (T3)

Brief Case Review

The usual age of diagnosis of schizophrenia is between the ages of 17 and 35. The common symptoms include hallucinations, delusions, disordered thinking, self-neglect, inappropriate emotions, and lack of emotions.

During the interview, the patient should be questioned regarding suicidal or homicidal ideations. If the person is thought to be a risk to himself/herself or to others, measures should be taken to avoid this. The patient should be referred for a full psychiatric evaluation and this should be conveyed to the caregiver as well as the patient during the interview. Drug screening should be done to rule out substance abuse as a cause of the symptoms. Alterations in thyroid hormone levels can result in psychiatric symptoms and therefore should be assayed.

CASE 14

Differential Diagnosis

1. *Migraine*
2. Trauma
3. Tension headache
4. Cluster headache
5. Subarachnoid aneurysm (rupture)
6. Temporal arteritis

Follow-Up

1. Computed tomography (CT) scan (if necessary)
2. Lumbar puncture (LP) (if necessary)

Brief Case Review

The common symptoms of a migraine headache include pain, nausea, vomiting, and sensitivity to lights and sounds. Some patients experience an aura prior to the onset of the migraine. Migraine headaches seem to have many triggers. Common triggers include certain foods, stress, hormonal changes, medications, and changes in the weather. The patient should be advised to avoid foods such as chocolate and dairy products and also to avoid alcohol and caffeine as these are common migraine triggers. A ruptured aneurysm also presents with a severe headache and is most common in this age group and so should be considered in the diagnosis. The most appropriate follow-up is to counsel the patient to avoid triggers such as certain foods, etc. If there is any doubt that this is a migraine headache, further investigations should be done. An LP can rule out a subarachnoid bleed or meningitis as a cause of the headache. A CT scan should also be considered.

CASE 15

Differential Diagnosis

1. *Domestic violence*
2. Syncope
3. Alcohol abuse
4. Drug abuse
5. Grand mal seizures
6. Psychosis

Follow-Up

1. Social worker's assessment of children's safety in the home
2. Toxicology (drug screening)
3. Electroencephalogram (EEG)

Brief Case Review

In a case such as this one, remember to investigate all types of violence occurring in the home. Domestic abuse can involve physical abuse, sexual abuse, and emotional abuse. Try to encourage the patient to discuss any problems or concerns that she may have. Reassuring the patient that the interview is confidential may be of value in this case. Assessing the overall safety of the individual is very important as well as the safety of any other persons residing in the home, such as children. The patient should be offered counseling and referred to support groups and help hotlines. She should also be made aware of domestic violence shelters in the area.

CASE 16

Differential Diagnosis

1. *Viral upper respiratory tract infection*
2. Pneumonia
3. Laryngotracheobronchitis
4. Anxiety
5. Foreign body aspiration

Follow-Up

1. Chest X-ray (CXR)
2. Spirometry
3. Pulmonary function testing (PFTs)
4. Complete blood count (CBC)
5. Sputum sample
6. Arterial blood gases (ABGs)

Brief Case Review

Common symptoms of asthma include cough, wheezing, shortness of breath, and chest tightness. Asthma is characterized by a combination of both bronchoconstriction as well as inflammation. Many triggers have been identified including dust, animal dander, viral infections, cold environments, smoke, and exercise. Although the patient in the case is a known asthmatic, underlying causes of the current asthma exacerbation must be investigated. A CBC and a sputum sample are useful for assessing the patient for an underlying infection. ABGs should be considered if the exacerbation is severe enough to warrant them.

CASE 17

Differential Diagnosis

1. *Gastric ulcer*
2. Colon cancer
3. Hemorrhoids
4. Vaginal bleeding
5. Colonic polyps

Follow-Up

1. Digital rectal examination (DRE)
2. Stool for occult blood
3. Complete blood count (CBC)
4. Esophagogastroduodenoscopy (EGD)
5. Colonoscopy
6. Blood group and cross match

Brief Case Review

There are many different causes of melena. These causes included upper GI causes, lower GI causes, and medication use. Upper GI bleeding tends to produce black, tarry stools. The partially digested blood is responsible for the appearance of the stool. Lower GI bleeding tends to produce either maroon-colored stool or bright red blood in the stool. Some common causes of upper GI bleeding to consider are gastric or duodenal ulcer, Mallory–Weiss tear, foreign body, trauma, and gastritis. Some common causes of lower GI bleeding are inflammatory bowel disease, colon cancer, hemorrhoids, intestinal infection, trauma, and colon polyps. Certain medications including iron supplements and bismuth can also cause black stool and should be considered in the diagnosis. In this case, the appearance of the stool combined with the patients other symptoms make medication an unlikely cause of the melena. Obtaining a complete social history is very important in this case as alcohol can predispose to conditions such as gastritis, Mallory–Weiss tears, and esophageal varices. The follow-up should include a CBC as this patients fatigue and dizziness may be due to hypovolemia resulting from blood loss. All GI bleeding should be considered a medical emergency.

CASE 18

Differential Diagnosis

1. *Type 2 diabetes mellitus*
2. *Type 1 diabetes mellitus*
3. Diabetes insipidus
4. Urinary tract infection (UTI)

Follow-Up

1. Blood glucose level
2. Glycosylated hemoglobin level (HgA1C)
3. Urinalysis (U/A)

Brief Case Review

Diabetes can occur in any age group and should be considered in any patient with complaints of weight loss and fatigue. Common symptoms of diabetes include polyuria, polydipsia, weight loss, fatigue, blurred vision, increased appetite, and slow healing infections. Long-term follow-up is necessary for patients with diabetes to monitor for complications. Nutritional counseling and education regarding the illness are key components of any treatment program. The patient should be educated about his illness and allowed to participate in decisions regarding his care. HgA1C should be done approximately every 3 months to assess glucose control.

CASE 19

Differential Diagnosis

1. *Carpal tunnel syndrome*
2. Tendonitis
3. Trauma
4. Sprain
5. Rheumatoid arthritis
6. Cervical spine disorder

Follow-Up

1. Wrist splint
2. Rheumatoid factor (RF)
3. Antinuclear factor (ANF)
4. Erythrocyte sedimentation rate (ESR)
5. Blood glucose level
6. Thyroid stimulating hormone (TSH)
7. Free thyroxine (T4)/free triiodothyroxine (T3)

8. Skull X-ray (if endocrine cause is suspected)
9. Beta human chorionic gonadotrophin (β-HCG) (if pregnancy is suspected)

Brief Case Review

Carpal tunnel commonly presents with tingling and numbness over the distribution of the median nerve. Women are more commonly affected compared to men and repetitive activity seems to be a risk factor for developing the condition. The condition is caused by compression of the median nerve as it passes under the flexor retinaculum. Remember that the structures that pass below the flexor retinaculum include the flexor tendons of the forearm muscles and the median nerve. Other than repetitive activities certain endocrine disorders such as acromegaly, diabetes mellitus, and thyroid disease can all predispose to the condition. Pregnancy and menopause are other conditions to consider. Inflammatory joint diseases such as rheumatoid arthritis and systemic lupus erythmatosus are also common causes of carpal tunnel syndrome; therefore, rheumatoid factor and antinuclear factor should be included in the follow-up.

CASE 20

Differential Diagnosis

1. *Gout*
2. Trauma
3. Osteomyelitis
4. Osteoarthritis
5. Stress fracture
6. Cellulitis

Follow-Up

1. Serum uric acid level
2. Joint aspiration and synovial fluid microscopy
3. X-ray (of affected joint)
4. Complete blood count (CBC)
5. Blood urea nitrogen level (BUN) and blood creatinine level
6. Lipid profile

Brief Case Review

The common symptoms of gout include pain, swelling, redness, and limited mobility of the affected joint. The most commonly affected joint is the first metatarsalphalangeal joint. Individuals who are at risk for developing gout include males, patients who use alcohol, patient's with diets rich in protein, and patients with exposure to lead. A family history of gout is usually present. An X-ray may be useful for differentiating gout from other causes of joint inflammation. A CBC may help to establish the presence of infection.

CASE 21

Differential Diagnosis

1. *Polycystic ovary disease*
2. Anorexia
3. Hyperthyroidism
4. Hyperprolactinemia
5. Stress/anxiety
6. Turner's syndrome
7. Chromosomal abnormality

Follow-Up

1. Bimanual pelvic examination
2. Breast examination
3. Complete blood count (CBC)
4. Prolactin level
5. Assessment of tubal patency
6. Chromosome analysis

Brief Case Review

Infertility is defined as the inability to conceive a child following one year of un-protected, regular intercourse. There are many causes of infertility and each of these should be explored thoroughly. There are many reasons that a couple may be infertile. These include an underlying medical problem in either the man or the woman as well as psychiatric problems affecting the woman. Stress, diet, and anxiety can all affect a woman's ability to conceive. Alcohol and cigarette use by either partner can have an influence on the couple's ability to achieve a pregnancy. The history should include a full history of the patient as well as a detailed history of her partner. Family history of psychiatric diseases is also im-portant to explore. The patient should be advised to have a follow-up visit with her partner. The prospect of counseling should be discussed with the patient.

CASE 22

Differential Diagnosis

1. *Bacterial dysentery*
2. Viral dysentery
3. Parasitic dysentery

4. Medication side effect
5. Colonic neoplasm

Follow-Up

1. Stool culture and examination for ova, cysts, and parasites
2. CD4+ cell count

Brief Case Review

AIDS is a retroviral disease, which allows the patient to become susceptible to a wide variety of opportunistic infections. Most AIDS patients experience diarrhea at some point. It is important to remember that due to the increased susceptibility of these patients to opportunistic infections all such infections must be considered. Included in your differential should be parasitic infections, viral infections, and bacterial infections. Diarrhea as a result of one of the current medications that the patient is taking must also be considered. Besides investigating the specifics regarding the diarrhea and eliciting any clinical signs, the patient should also be counseled prior to the end of the session. Patient education and encouraging both the use of continuing current medication as well as encouraging the patient to practice safe sex are a vital part of the interview. The risk of transmission to other individuals through sexual contact, contact with bodily fluids, shared needles, and so on should be discussed. Also discuss possible risks of transmission through occupation, sports, accidents, and so forth.

CASE 23

Differential Diagnosis

1. *Gonorrhea*
2. Chlamydia

3. Urinary tract infection (UTI)
4. Pyelonephritis
5. Appendicitis

Follow-Up

1. Urethral culture
2. Urinalysis (U/A)
3. Urine culture
4. Complete blood count (CBC)

Brief Case Review

Common symptoms of gonorrhea in males include dysuria, a greenish-yellowish penile discharge and occasionally swollen or painful testicles. Some men may remain asymptomatic. Many women remain asymptomatic. Some women experience symptoms, which include dysuria, vaginal discharge, vaginal bleeding in-between periods. Women can develop PID from untreated infection; therefore, early diagnosis is important. In men, untreated cases can lead to epididymitis, which can eventually lead to sterility.

CASE 24

Differential Diagnosis

1. *Medial collateral ligament tear*
2. Anterior cruciate ligament tear
3. Medial meniscus tear
4. Dislocation
5. Fracture

Follow-Up

1. X-ray
2. Magnetic resonance imaging (MRI)

Brief Case Review

Knee injuries are common injuries incurred by soccer players. Remember the unhappy triad: ACL, MCL, and medial meniscus. A detailed account of the accident is an important part of the history as this will give insight to the injury received. A full knee examination should be performed to assess all of the ligaments of the knee. An X-ray can help to rule out a fracture or a dislocation and an MRI is useful for evaluating a torn ligament.

CASE 25

Differential Diagnosis

1. *Tuberculosis*
2. Pneumonia
3. Lung abscess
4. Bronchitis
5. Aspiration of gastric contents

Follow-Up

1. Respiratory isolation
2. Tuberculin skin test (PPD)

3. Chest X-ray (CXR)
4. Sputum culture
5. HIV test
6. Computed tomography (CT) scan
7. Bronchoscopy
8. Alcohol withdrawal precautions

Brief Case Review

Common symptoms of tuberculosis include cough, hemoptysis, fever, night sweats, weight loss, fatigue, shortness of breath, and chest pain. The incidence of tuberculosis is on the rise and should be considered in any patient with a cough, particularly when associated with weight loss and hemoptysis. Patients living in crowded living situations are at increased risk of tuberculosis. The patient in the case has an increased risk of contracting tuberculosis because of both his living situation and his problem with alcohol abuse. The placement of a PPD along with a CXR are invaluable in this case. The patient should be counseled regarding the use of alcohol and advised to seek help in order to stop drinking. AIDS should always be considered as an underlying risk factor for tuberculosis.

CASE 26

Differential Diagnosis

1. *Rheumatoid arthritis*
2. Osteoarthritis
3. Systemic lupus erythematosus
4. Bursitis
5. Tendonitis
6. Hepatitis

Follow-Up

1. X-rays of affected joints
2. Rheumatoid factor (RF)
3. Erythrocyte sedimentation rate (ESR)
4. Joint aspiration and synovial fluid microscopy
5. Complete blood count (CBC)

Brief Case Review

The most likely diagnosis in this case is rheumatoid arthritis. Common symptoms of rheumatoid arthritis and other inflammatory arthritides such as systemic lupus erythematosus (SLE) include pain and swelling of the joints, morning stiffness, decreased mobility of the affected joints, and fatigue. Rheumatoid arthritis typically affects the smaller joints of the body. In particular, the hands, wrists, feet, and the knees. Osteoarthritis should be considered in the differential; however, osteoarthritis does not have the classic, prolonged morning stiffness and more commonly affects the larger joints of the body such as the hips.

CASE 27

Differential Diagnosis

1. *Primary enuresis*
2. Urinary tract infection (UTI)
3. Diabetes mellitus
4. Congenital abnormality of the urinary tract

Follow-Up

1. Full physical examination
2. Urinalysis (U/A)
3. Urine culture
4. Enuresis alarm
5. Ultrasound

Brief Case Review

Enuresis affects many children. There are many different causes of enuresis. Underlying causes such as a UTI should be investigated. Emotional instability, stress, and heredity also seem to play a role in bed wetting. In this case, once underlying causes have been ruled out, behavior modification such as the use of an enuresis alarm is the next step. The father should be advised not to discipline his son regarding this matter as this can aggravate the problem. The father should also be reassured that this is a common problem and that most children eventually outgrow this without any intervention.

CASE 28

Differential Diagnosis

1. *Normal grief*
2. Depression
3. Rheumatoid arthritis
4. Osteoarthritis
5. Hypothyroidism

6. Bipolar disorder
7. Alcohol abuse
8. Drug abuse
9. Anemia

Follow-Up

1. Rheumatoid factor (RF)
2. X-rays of affected joints
3. Thyroid stimulating hormone (TSH)
4. Free thyroxine (T4)/free triiodothyroxine (T3)
5. Complete blood count (CBC)
6. Toxicology (drug screening)

Brief Case Review

Although this patient's symptoms are most likely secondary to his grief, underlying pathology must still be suspected and fully investigated. It is very important to assess the patient's support system. His ability to function without his wife will also need to be assessed. Encourage the patient to try to participate in activities he enjoys, such as his twice weekly card games with his friends. Allow the patient to talk openly and freely during the interview about any feelings and emotions that he may be experiencing. Suggest that the patient start counseling and encourage his attendance at support groups.

CASE 29

Differential Diagnosis

1. *Essential hypertension*
2. Renal disease
3. Pheochromocytoma
4. Primary aldosteronism
5. Cocaine abuse

Follow-Up

1. Urinalysis (U/A)
2. Lipid profile
3. 24-hour urinary catecholamines and metanephrines
4. Renal ultrasound
5. Computed tomography (CT) scan
6. Toxicology (drug screening)

Brief Case Review

Common symptoms of hypertension include headache, blurred vision, dizziness, and palpitations. Unfortunately, most hypertensive patients do not actually experience any symptoms from their increased blood pressure. This leads to a lot of undiagnosed cases. There are many causes of hypertension, the most common being essential hypertension with no identifiable underlying cause. Patients with hypertension require frequent office visits to ensure that their blood pressure is being well controlled. Patient education is very important as many hypertensive patients can be managed without the use of medications. Counseling regarding healthy lifestyle choices should be included as part of any encounter. The patient should be advised to stop smoking if relevant, lose weight if necessary, decrease salt intake, increase vegetables in diet, and exercise regularly.

CASE 30

Differential Diagnosis

1. *Urinary tract infection* (UTI)
2. Pyelonephritis
3. Vaginitis
4. Pelvic inflammatory disease
5. Appendicitis
6. Herpes simplex type 2

Follow-Up

1. Urinalysis (U/A)
2. Urine culture
3. Bimanual pelvic examination
4. Vaginal cultures
5. Complete blood count (CBC)

Brief Case Review

Common symptoms of a UTI include dysuria, urgency, frequency, and pelvic pain. Patients may also notice that their urine has a foul odor and in some cases there may be hematuria. Patients with pyelonephritis typically have the same complaints but generally also complain of fever and flank pain. STDs and PID need to be considered in any young sexually active female with abdominal pain.

CASE 31

Differential Diagnosis

1. *Hyperthyroidism*
2. Anxiety disorder
3. Bipolar disorder
4. Anorexia nervosa/bulimia
5. Intestinal parasitosis
6. Drug (cocaine) abuse

Follow-Up

1. Thyroid stimulating hormone (TSH)
2. Free thyroxine (T4)/free triiodothyroxine (T3)
3. Ultrasound of the thyroid gland
4. Stool culture and stool for ova, cysts, and parasites
5. Radionuclide uptake scan of the thyroid gland
6. Toxicology (drug screening)

Brief Case Review

Common symptoms of hyperthyroidism include weight loss, anxiety, tremors, palpitations, diarrhea, and a change in menstrual periods. In any individual presenting with anxiety, nervousness, tremors, etc., drug use must be ruled out as a cause of the symptoms. Psychiatric problems must also be considered as many of the symptoms common to hyperthyroidism can also be caused by psychiatric disorders. In any patient presenting with diarrhea and weight loss, a stool sample should be collected to rule out a parasitic infection.

CASE 32

Differential Diagnosis

1. *Appendicitis*
2. Urinary tract infection (UTI)
3. Pelvic inflammatory disease (female)
4. Ectopic pregnancy (female)
5. Ovarian cyst (female)
6. Ovarian torsion (female)
7. Cholecystitis
8. Gastroenteritis
9. Viral disease with pelvic lymphadenitis

Follow-Up

1. Digital rectal examination (DRE)
2. Beta human chorionic gonadotrophin (β-HCG) (female)
3. Pelvic examination (female)
4. Complete blood count (CBC)
5. Urinalysis (U/A)]
6. Pelvic/abdominal ultrasound

Brief Case Review

The most likely diagnosis in this case is appendicitis given the symptoms as well as the age of the patient. Most commonly affected are individuals in the second and third decades of life. Males are more often affected compared to females. The classic presentation of appendicitis is pain initially located around the umbilicus, which later moves to the right lower quadrant. Fever, nausea, vomiting, and anorexia are generally early symptoms. In this case, it is very important to consider other causes of female abdominal pain including ectopic pregnancy. A pregnancy test should be performed regardless of the patient's stated LMP.

CASE 33

Differential Diagnosis

Smoking cessation

Follow-Up

Counseling

Brief Case Review

The most important aspect of this patient encounter is counseling. In this case, if possible the patient's wife should also be encouraged to quit smoking.

CASE 34

Differential Diagnosis

1. *Hemorrhoids*
2. Anal fissure
3. Colon polyps
4. Diverticulosis
5. Dilverticulitis
6. Colon cancer

Follow-Up

1. Digital rectal examination (DRE)
2. Stool guiac
3. Complete blood count (CBC)
4. Sigmoidoscopy
5. Colonoscopy

Brief Case Review

There are many different causes of hematochezia. Two common and fairly benign causes to be considered are hemorrhoids and anal fissures. A detailed history of the bleeding should be obtained. It is important to ascertain the color of the blood and the location of the blood (i.e., toilet paper vs. in the stool itself). Other symptoms of hemorrhoids and anal fissures are rectal discomfort, itching, and rectal burning. In this case the patient is worried about the possibility of polyps and celiac disease. This patient should have a colonoscopy regardless. Colonoscopy should be offered as a routine part of health care maintenance to all individuals over the age of 50. This patient warrants a colonoscopy because of both his age and his symptoms. It is unlikely that the patient has celiac disease as he has had no weight loss and celiac disease generally presents at a much younger age. Steatorrhea is generally present in patients with celiac disease rather than hematochezia.

CASE 35

Differential Diagnosis

1. *Unstable angina*
2. Myocardial infarction
3. Coronary artery spasm
4. Pleuritis
5. Pneumonia
6. Musculoskeletal pain
7. Trauma

Follow-Up

1. Electrocardiogram (ECG)
2. Cardiac enzymes (CK, CK-MB, Troponin)
3. Chest X-ray (CXR)
4. Echocardiogram (EcHO)
5. Stress test
6. Lipid profile
7. Counseling for smoking cessation

Brief Case Review

See Case 38 (stable angina). In this case the patient should be counseled regarding smoking cessation prior to the end of the interview.

CASE 36

Differential Diagnosis

1. *Cocaine abuse*
2. Alcohol abuse
3. Depression
4. HIV
5. Anxiety
6. Hyperthyroidism
7. Anemia

Follow-Up

1. Evaluate HIV status
2. Thyroid stimulating hormone (TSH)
3. Free thyroxine (T4)/free triiodothyroxine (T3)
4. Complete blood count (CBC)
5. Liver function tests (LFTs)

Brief Case Review

Cocaine is an addictive, illegal, stimulant drug. Its effects on the body include increased heart rate, increased blood pressure, increased temperature, increased energy, irritability, auditory hallucinations, restlessness, and dilated pupils. Other effects of cocaine include chest pain, arrhythmias, strokes, seizures, and respiratory failure. One of the most important issues to address in a case such as this one is the patient's emotional well-being. Assess the patient carefully for signs of depression and any suicidal thoughts. The patient should be counseled during the interview as to the effects of cocaine and alcohol use and long-term counseling should be discussed.

CASE 37

Differential Diagnosis

1. *Sickle-cell crisis*
2. Drug-seeking behavior
3. Pneumonia
4. Rib fracture
5. Costochondritis
6. Anxiety

Follow-Up

1. Complete blood count (CBC)
2. Urinalysis (U/A)
3. Electrolytes
4. Chest X-ray

Brief Case Review

Sickle-cell anemia is inherited as an autosomal recessive trait. An important aspect of the history in this case is to establish other members of the family who have either the disease or the trait. Common symptoms of painful crisis in sickle-cell disease are chest pain, abdominal pain, fatigue, breathlessness, jaundice, fever, and delayed growth. Recurrent painful crises can result in damage to the kidneys, lungs, eyes, central nervous system, and bones. Unfortunately, because of the need for narcotics many of these patients develop tolerance and addiction to these drugs. Drug-seeking behavior must be considered in these patients. A U/A should be performed as part of the follow-up to assess for urinary casts or the presence of hematuria. CXR may be useful to rule out pneumonia or rib fracture as a cause of the chest pain. The patient should be counseled with regards to a healthy lifestyle. Triggers should be identified and avoided in the future.

CASE 38

Differential Diagnosis

1. *Stable angina*
2. Myocardial infarction
3. Pleuritis
4. Pneumonia
5. Musculoskeletal pain
6. Trauma

Follow-Up

1. Electrocardiogram (ECG)
2. Cardiac enzymes (CK, CK-MB, Troponin)

3. Chest X-ray (CXR)
4. Echocardiogram (EcHO)
5. Stress test
6. Lipid profile

Brief Case Review

There are three types of angina: stable, unstable, and Prinzmetal's (variant) angina. Patients with stable angina experience pain with exertion which is relieved with medication, and patients with unstable angina experience pain both with exertion or at rest and the pain is not relieved with medication. Patients with Prinzmetal's experience pain at rest (particularly in the early morning) which is relieved with medication. Patients experiencing any form of angina require extensive cardiac testing. Musculoskeletal pain should always be considered in any patient with chest pain. A complete history and a detailed physical examination should be performed to rule this out.

CASE 39

Differential Diagnosis

1. *Pregnancy*
2. Polycystic ovary disease

Follow-Up

1. Bimanual pelvic examination
2. Beta human chorionic gonadotrophin (β-HCG) (female)
3. Abdominal ultrasound

4. Complete blood count (CBC)
5. Urinalysis (U/A)
6. Vaginal cultures
7. Blood group
8. Venereal disease research laboratory (VDRL)
9. HIV test

Brief Case Review

In a case such as this one, a complete history is vital. The patient's past obstetric history including outcomes of previous pregnancies is very important. The other aspect of the history, which is very important, is any current or past history of the patient herself and also a family history of any diseases (particularly genetic disorders). The patient should be advised about lifestyle changes such as diet, exercise, smoking, alcohol, and drug use. In this case, the patient is reportedly happy about the prospect of being pregnant; however, this may not always be the case. In a case where there is an unwanted pregnancy, counseling regarding the patient's options should be done. There are numerous routine blood tests performed during a pregnancy, these include VDRL, HIV, blood group, and a CBC.

CASE 40

Differential Diagnosis

1. *Pneumonia*
2. Tuberculosis
3. Lung abscess
4. Bronchitis
5. Bronchiectasis

Follow-Up

1. Chest X-ray (CXR)
2. Sputum culture
3. Tuberculin skin test (PPD)
4. Computed tomography (CT) scan
5. Bronchoscopy

Brief Case Review

Common symptoms of pneumonia include cough (usually productive of greenish/yellow sputum), fever, chest pain, shortness of breath, and fatigue. Often persons with limited mobility or disabilities are more prone to developing pneumonia, which may be a factor in this case. Tuberculosis must always be considered in any patient with a cough and a PPD test should be performed to rule this out.

CASE 41

Differential Diagnosis

1. *Alcoholic neuropathy*
2. Diabetic neuropathy
3. Cerebrovascular accident
4. Vascular insufficiency
5. Toxic neuropathy
6. Carpal tunnel syndrome (hand involvement only)

Follow-Up

1. Liver function tests (LFTs)
2. Protime/prothrombin time (PT/PTT)
3. Ultrasound of the liver
4. Blood glucose level
5. Complete blood count (CBC)
6. Doppler studies
7. Electromyography (EMG)

Brief Case Review

Symptoms of alcoholic neuropathy include numbness, muscle weakness, paresthesias, heat intolerance, difficulty urinating, diarrhea, vomiting, as well as numerous other symptoms. Given the patient's history of alcohol abuse in this case, alcoholic neuropathy is the most likely diagnosis. Factors to consider when deciding appropriate follow-up for this patient are other complications associated with long-term alcohol use. Liver function tests as well as an assessment of the patient's nutritional status are both very important in this case. A proper assessment of mental status is also appropriate in this case as the patient may have developed Wernicke–Korsakoff's syndrome. EMG may be a useful tool to evaluate the degree of the neurological damage.

CASE 42

Differential Diagnosis

1. *Hypothyroidism*
2. Depression
3. Bipolar disorder

4. Lithium therapy
5. Anemia

Follow-Up

1. Thyroid stimulating hormone (TSH)
2. Free thyroxine (T4)/free triiodothyroxine (T3)
3. Ultrasound of the thyroid gland
4. Complete blood count (CBC)

Brief Case Review

Common symptoms of hypothyroidism include weight gain, constipation, fatigue, depression, mental slowing, and changes in menstrual periods. The symptoms of hypothyroidism may be vague and mild and the condition can often go undiagnosed for a long period of time. Often times the patient attributes all of the symptoms to depression and does not seek medical care. Psychiatric disorders should be considered in any patient complaining of symptoms such as fatigue, lethargy, depression, and weight gain. Patients being treated with lithium often experience many of the symptoms common to hypothyroidism. This should be taken into consideration and a complete drug history should be taken. Anemia can also cause many of the symptoms common to hypothyroidism and can be ruled out by a simple CBC.

CASE 43

Differential Diagnosis

1. *Lung cancer*
2. Tuberculosis
3. Pneumonia
4. Lung abscess
5. Bronchitis

Follow-Up

1. Chest X-ray (CXR)
2. Sputum culture
3. Tuberculin skin test (PPD)
4. Computed tomography (CT) scan
5. Bronchoscopy

Brief Case Review

Common symptoms of lung cancer include cough, hemoptysis, dyspnea, weight loss, fatigue, and chest pain. Most lung cancers are secondary to cigarette smoking. In this case, tuberculosis should be high on the differential as many of the symptoms are common to both pathologies. CXR is very useful in this case as it can be used to differentiate between lung cancer, tuberculosis, and pneumonia. During the interview, the patient should also be counseled regarding smoking cessation.

CASE 44

Differential Diagnosis

1. *Viral meningitis*
2. Bacterial meningitis
3. Encephalitis
4. Migraine
5. Tension headache

Follow-Up

1. Lumbar puncture (LP)
2. Complete blood count (CBC)
3. Blood culture
4. Computed tomography (CT) scan

Brief Case Review

Common symptoms of meningitis include headache, fever, nausea, vomiting, nuchal rigidity, and altered mental status. The most important diagnostic test in this case is an LP. An LP can differentiate between bacterial meningitis and viral meningitis. A proper opthalmoscopic examination should precede an LP since a finding of papilloedema would make an LP hazardous. There are many other causes of headaches and all of these must be taken into consideration. In a case such as this one in which meningitis is the likely diagnosis, patient isolation should be considered.

CASE 45

Differential Diagnosis

1. *Depression*
2. Hypothyroidism
3. Bipolar disorder
4. Alcohol abuse
5. Drug abuse
6. Diabetes mellitus
7. Anemia

Follow-Up

1. Thyroid stimulating hormone (TSH)
2. Free thyroxine (T4)/free triiodothyroxine (T3)
3. Toxicology (drug screening)
4. Fasting blood glucose level
5. Complete blood count (CBC)

Brief Case Review

Common symptoms of depression include tearfulness, feelings of worthlessness, decreased interest in activities/hobbies, increased or decreased appetite, early morning awakenings, decreased energy, difficulty concentrating, suicidal thoughts, and suicide attempts. It is important to rule out an underlying pathology as the cause of the symptoms. Hypothyroidism, diabetes, and anemia can all be ruled out by simple blood tests. Drug and alcohol abuse should be considered regardless of the history obtained from the patient. The patient should be asked about any suicidal thoughts or suicidal plans he/she may have. During the interview, counseling and support groups should be discussed and the patient should be encouraged to become involved in both.

CASE 46

CASE 46

Differential Diagnosis

1. *Gastric ulcer*
2. Hiatus hernia
3. Gastroesophageal reflux
4. Alcoholic gastritis
5. Acute on chronic pancreatitis
6. Gastric neoplasm
7. Esophageal spasm
8. Angina

Follow-Up

1. Digital rectal examination (DRE)
2. Stool guiac
3. Complete blood count (CBC)
4. Esophagogastroduodenoscopy (EGD)
5. Serum amylase
6. Serum lipase
7. *Helicobacter pylori* antibody test (blood test)
8. *Helicobacter pylori* breath test
9. Electrocardiogram (ECG)

Brief Case Review

Common symptoms of a gastric ulcer include epigastric pain, nausea, vomiting, weight loss, melena, and fatigue. Risk factors include *Helicobacter* infection, the use of non-steroidal anti-inflammatory drugs (NSAIDs), smoking, and alcohol use. Stool guiac and CBC are essential components of the follow-up to establish if the patient is having any GI bleeding. A detailed history along with an ECG can rule out angina as a cause of the chest pain in this case.

CASE 47

Differential Diagnosis

1. *Infectious mononucleosis*
2. Group A streptococcus (strep throat)
3. Influenza virus
4. Rhinovirus
5. Gingivitis

Follow-Up

1. Monospot test
2. Epstein–Barr virus antigen
3. Rapid strep test
4. Throat culture

Brief Case Review

Common symptoms of infectious mononucleosis (mono) include fever, sore throat, lymphadenopathy, and fatigue. The patient may also experience headache, muscle aches, drowsiness, cough, shortness of breath, and rash. Mono is typically transmitted through saliva so inquiring about ill contacts is an important part of the history. Other causes of sore throat must be considered including the common cold and strep throat. A proper abdominal examination to assess for splenomegaly should be done and the patient should be counseled to avoid contact sports as splenic rupture can occur with this infection.

CASE 48

Differential Diagnosis

1. *Palpitations*
2. Anxiety
3. Fever
4. Caffeine/nicotine use
5. Hyperthyroidism
6. Anemia
7. Mitral valve prolapse
8. Electrolyte imbalance

Follow-Up

1. Electrocardiogram (ECG)
2. Echocardiogram (EcHO)

3. Holter monitor
4. Complete blood count (CBC)
5. Thyroid stimulating hormone (TSH)
6. Free thyroxine (T4)/free triiodothyroxine (T3)
7. Electrolytes

Brief Case Review

There are many causes of palpitations. Some common causes include fever, stress, anxiety, medications, anemia, hyperventilation, caffeine use, nicotine use, hypoglycemia, hyperthyroidism, and certain pathological conditions. Heart conditions which may be the underling cause of palpitations include aortic stenosis, atrial fibrillation, mitral valve prolapse, premature ventricular contractions, and paroxysmal atrial tachycardia. An ECG should be included in the follow-up of any patient whose primary complaint is related to the heart. In this case, an EcHO should also be performed to rule out valve disease as the cause of the patient's symptoms. Simple blood tests can rule out anemia, hyperthyroidism, hypoglycemia, and electrolye imbalance.

CASE 49

Differential Diagnosis

1. *Concussion*
2. Grand mal seizure
3. Postural hypotension
4. Diabetes mellitus
5. Substance abuse

6. Anemia
7. Pregnancy
8. Intracranial mass

Follow-Up

1. Head X-ray
2. Computed tomography (CT) scan
3. Electroencephalogram (EEG)
4. Orthostatic blood pressures
5. Fasting blood glucose level
6. Electrocardiogram (ECG)
7. Beta human chorionic gonadotrophin (β-HCG) (female)
8. Complete blood count (CBC)
9. Toxicology (drug screening)

Brief Case Review

The classic symptoms of concussion include dizziness, confusion, headache, amnesia, loss of consciousness, nausea, vomiting, irritability, and difficulty concentrating. There are many causes of loss of consciousness in a young individual, which have to be ruled. In a young menstruating female, one major consideration is iron deficiency anemia. The patient should be assessed for postural hypotension and a CBC should be included as part of the follow-up. The patient should also be given a pregnancy test as part of the follow-up and drug screening should be carried out regardless of the history obtained from the patient. X-ray and CT should be performed to rule out skull fracture or intracranial bleeding as a cause of the symptoms.

CASE 50

Differential Diagnosis

1. *Menopause*
2. Pregnancy

Follow-Up

1. Bimanual pelvic examination
2. Beta human chorionic gonadotrophin (β-HCG) (female)
3. Abdominal ultrasound
4. Follicle stimulating hormone (FSH) level

Brief Case Review

Most women experience menopause between the ages of 48 and 55 with the average age being 51. The common symptoms that women experience include mood swings, hot flashes, difficulty sleeping, irregular periods or amenorrhea, and weight gain. In any woman with amenorrhea and who is also sexually active, pregnancy should be considered regardless of the patient's age. Counseling is an important aspect of the interview. Healthy lifestyle changes should be emphasized to decrease the chances of the patient developing osteoporosis. These include decreasing alcohol intake, quitting smoking, if relevant, eating a healthy diet, and regular exercise. FSH levels may be increased at the time of menopause and can be tested. Remember that FSH levels alone are not a reliable indicator of menopause and the diagnosis should be mainly based on symptoms.

CASE 51

Differential Diagnosis

1. *Cataracts*
2. Macular degeneration
3. Glaucoma
4. Presbyopia
5. Alcohol use
6. Diabetic retinopathy
7. Medication side effect

Follow-Up

1. Stronger glasses or bifocals
2. Recommend appropriate lighting in home
3. Blood glucose level
4. Serum calcium

Brief Case Review

Cataracts commonly cause blurred vision, increased difficulty with night vision, halos around lights or objects, and fading of colors. The onset of the symptoms is generally gradual and painless. Cataracts are caused by clouding or opacities of the lens of the eye. They generally occur in the older population or following a traumatic injury to the eye. Certain conditions predispose an individual to develop cataracts and these include diabetes, previous history of cataracts, smoking, previous eye surgery, prolonged use of corticosteroids, and rarely parathyroid disease. The only real cure for cataracts is surgery; however, some measures may be taken to assist the patient. These include adequate lighting in the home, the use of magnifying glasses for reading as needed, and limited night driving.

CASE 52

Differential Diagnosis

1. *Benign prostatic hyperplasia*
2. Renal calculi
3. Bladder calculi
4. Trauma
5. Medication use
6. Bladder cancer
7. Renal cancer
8. Urinary tract infection (UTI)

Follow-Up

1. Digital rectal examination (DRE)
2. Genital examination
3. Urinalysis (U/A)
4. Urine cytology
5. Prostate specific antigen (PSA)
6. Cystoscopy
7. Intravenous pyelogram (IVP)

Brief Case Review

There are many causes of hematuria. First it must be established that the patient is actually experiencing hematuria. This can be done by a simple U/A. There are numerous causes of pseudohematuria including excessive consumption of berries, rhubarb, and beets. Also there are many medications that can cause the urine to appear reddish/brown. A DRE should be performed to assess the prostate gland. If no cause for the hematuria can be found, then the patient should undergo cystoscopy and IVP.

CASE 53

Differential Diagnosis

1. *Pelvic inflammatory disease*
2. Appendicitis
3. Meckel's diverticulitis
4. Ectopic pregnancy
5. Urinary tract infection (UTI)

Follow-Up

1. Bimanual pelvic examination
2. Vaginal cultures
3. Complete blood count (CBC)
4. Abdominal ultrasound
5. Beta human chorionic gonadotrophin (β-HCG)
6. Urinalysis (U/A)
7. Urine culture

Brief Case Review

Common symptoms of pelvic inflammatory disease include abdominal/pelvic pain, vaginal discharge, fever, nausea, vomiting, and dyspareunia. Complications of PID include infertility and an increased risk of ectopic pregnancy. The patient should have vaginal cultures taken. A pregnancy test should be done to rule out the possibility that the abdominal pain is due to an ectopic pregnancy. UTI is always a consideration in a young female with abdominal pain and should be tested for.

CASE 54

Differential Diagnosis

1. *Anxiety/Depression*
2. Erectile dysfunction secondary to diabetes
3. Drug use
4. Multiple sclerosis
5. Tertiary syphilis

Follow-Up

1. Genital examination
2. Diabetes management
3. Blood glucose level
4. Glycosylated hemoglobin (HgA1C)
5. Venereal Disease Research Laboratory (VDRL)

Brief Case Review

Impotence is a very sensitive issue to deal with. Open-ended questions are a key component to the interview and will allow the patient to express his concerns and anxieties. It is very important to differentiate between erectile dysfunction due to psychogenic causes and erectile dysfunction due to an underlying disease. If the patient is continuing to have early morning erections or erections at other times, then the cause is more likely to be psychological. If the patient is never experiencing erections, then the cause is more likely to be due to an underlying disease. There are many conditions which can lead to impotence, common ones include diabetes, multiple sclerosis, syphilis, all of which should be ruled out as part of the work-up. Treatment is going to be largely based on the underlying cause of the impotence. During the interview, the patient should be counseled regarding the care and management of his diabetes.

CASE 55

Differential Diagnosis

1. *Ectopic pregnancy*
2. Pelvic inflammatory disease (female)
3. Appendicitis
4. Ovarian cyst (female)
5. Ovarian torsion (female)
6. Urinary tract infection (UTI)

Follow-Up

1. Bimanual pelvic examination
2. Beta human chorionic gonadotrophin (β-HCG) (female)

3. Vaginal cultures
4. Abdominal ultrasound
5. Complete blood count (CBC)
6. Urinalysis (U/A)

Brief Case Review

Common symptoms of an ectopic pregnancy include abdominal/pelvic pain, nausea, amenorrhea, breast tenderness, and vaginal bleeding. The most common site of an ectopic pregnancy is in the ampulla of the fallopian tube. Risk factors include a history of PID, prior surgery, a previous ectopic pregnancy, endometriosis, the presence of adhesions or scar tissue, or the use of an intrauterine device (IUD). It is therefore very important to obtain a very detailed and complete sexual/obstetric history of the patient. A β-HCG should be performed in any female with abdominal pain regardless of the patient's sexual history or the date of the last menstrual period. Abdominal ultrasound may be useful in differentiating an ectopic pregnancy from an ovarian cyst or ovarian torsion.

Case Index